TRIUMPH
OVER
DARKNESS

Understanding and Healing
the Trauma of Childhood Sexual Abuse

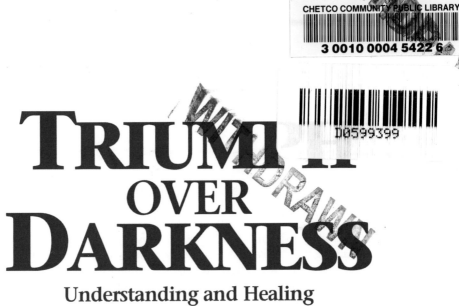

Wendy Ann Wood, M.A.

Foreword by
Marilyn Van Derbur
former Miss America and incest survivor

Chetco Community Public Library
405 Alder Street
Brookings, OR 97415

Published by Beyond Words Publishing, Inc.
13950 N.W. Pumpkin Ridge Road
Hillsboro, OR 97123
Phone: (503) 647-5109
Toll Free: 1-800-284-9673
Fax: (503) 647-5114

The poems, letters, journal entries, and other accounts in this collection were sent to the author to be published as recovery readings on incest, rape, and abuse. In the interests of privacy, contributors' names have been changed or abbreviated.

Printed by Friesen Printers in Canada
Distributed by Publishers Group West

Editor: Julie Livingston
Jacket design: Gary Lund
First printing: April,1988

Library of Congress Cataloging-in-Publication Data

Wood, Wendy Ann, 1953-
    Triumph over darkness : understanding and healing the trauma of childhood sexual abuse / Wendy Ann Wood : foreword by Marilyn Van Derbur
        p.   cm.
    "First printing April, 1988"—Verso t.p.
    Includes bibliographical references.
    ISBN 0-941831-86-8 : $12.95
    1. Adult child sexual abuse victims   I. Title.
RC569.5.A28W66   1993
616.85′822390651—dc20   93-18381
                                                                CIP

This book was written in loving memory
of my mother, Marjory D. Wood. She taught me
the meaning of living and life and was the
wind beneath my wings — my silver thread.
She is greatly missed

It is dedicated to you, the survivor,
as you journey your own path of healing.

CONTENTS

Acknowledgments vi

Foreword viii

Introduction 1

Chapter 1 Echoes From The Darkness 17

Chapter 2 Seeing The Darkness Before The Light 51

Chapter 3 Moving Beyond The Darkness 91

Chapter 4 Voices Of Ritual Abuse Survivors 127

Chapter 5 Voices Of Male Survivors 163

Chapter 6 Voices Of Multiplicity 189

Chapter 7 Partners In Healing .207

Chapter 8 The Healing Process .225

Appendix 259

ACKNOWLEDGMENTS

I would like to thank my best friend, Leslie Hatton, who co-authored the first edition of this book with me. Leslie has put aside her writing life to deal with being a widow and raising her two young boys, Ryan and Daniel. Thank you for the encouragement to go it alone with this edition — you were missed, my friend. Maybe in a few years, when the boys go off to school, we can write together once again.

To my family — my dad, Carl, Doug and Gisela, Chip and Sharon — who have supported me unconditionally through the roller coaster ride life sometimes brings, I give my appreciation and love.

Thank you to my clients, whose strength and courage to pursue recovery continues to amaze me each day I work with you. Thank you for your wisdom and willingness to tell me that works and what doesn't, and the courage to have your voices heard in the questionnaires, workshops, and conferences you participated in. But mostly, thank you for letting me have the unique opportunity of walking beside you in your recovery journey. I believe in you all and in your potential for recovery.

I am grateful to Janice Dennison, my sister — not of blood or marriage but of the heart — who taught me the value of true friendship with her unconditional love and support, late night phone calls, and our lengthy conversations about recovery issues while we sat in my car. And my gratitude to her husband, Jack, my business manager, who has helped me maintain my growing business, thus allowing me the freedom to do the work I love most: counseling and writing.

Thanks to Christine Hatcher-Holte, another sister of the heart: someone who was there from the inception of the original *Triumph* at Echoes Counseling Center, and now for this edition. Your intellect, openness, sensitivity, centeredness — and oh yes, your willingness to share Lars and Noah with me — were so valuable.

I would like to thank Julie Livingston, my editor at Beyond Words Publishing, who held the light for me on this revised edition journey. Julie matched my pace with wonderful intuition and shared in the vision, the excitement, and the commitment to quality. Thank you does not adequately express my gratitude.

To Cindy Black and Richard Cohn, my publishers: It has been a real joy to see us all grow older and wiser together. We do get better with age, don't we! Richard pulled the original manuscript of *Triumph* out of our closets and produced the reality of our vision. Cindy provided me with the encouragement and inspiration to visualize this edition and beyond it.

To Susan Jacobs, an Awalt High School English teacher, who entered my life for a few brief semesters some twenty-odd years ago to teach me the true value of journaling and self-discovery: Please get in touch with me — I want to say thank you in person.

A special thanks to Kurt Ruttman, who maintains his commitment to the cause of recovery from childhood sexual abuse by giving his time and counsel on the legal aspects of this problem.

Lifetime support people mean so much, to which this book attests. My acknowledgments would not be complete without mentioning Franzi Corman, Scott Trusdale, Brian Posewitz, Janet Brown-Coggins, Lori Jolly-McWeithy, and Norma Gayton; also Dennis, Karen, and Jamie Marceaux; Etta Marie Schaffer; Joyce Cantrell, M.D.; and Nancy and Jim Clark. For the support people who have left my life over the years, there are pieces of my heart missing.

Finally, this book would never have come about were it not for the brave, insightful, and creative contributors whose stories are bound within these pages. These survivors live all over the world. Some I have had the pleasure to meet, know, and/or talk with on the phone. Most are people whom I feel I have known forever, though I have only met them through the mail. Thank you all for opening your lives to me so that the pages of this book could unfold.

And to Corry and Heidi, I say, "Let's go to the beach!"

FOREWORD

It has been a more than a year since I first spoke the words, but I was fifty-three years old before I was able to say, "My name is Marilyn Van Derbur Atler, and I am an incest survivor."

Through my correspondence with over 5,000 survivors, I am beginning to understand that recovery is a manageable, predictable process. If you are still locked into the horrific shame, if you are still suffering from the emotional and physical traumas of your childhood, I say to you, THE PAIN ENDS! I promise you — *if* you do your work. There are no short cuts. No surgeon can open you up and remove your shame and pain. Only through speaking, telling your story, can healing begin.

Some of our friends and family members think we are having a total nervous breakdown. We are not. We are going through recovery. Just as a person who has suffered a heart attack would be placed in an intensive care unit, survivors of sexual abuse need intensive care because our hearts were broken. Anger, grief, rage, despair, hopelessness — all of these feelings are normal, just as being bedridden and hooked up to an I.V. is normal for a heart attack survivor.

Recovery was a long and agonizing process for me. There were days when I knew I would have to die — not because I wanted to, but because I couldn't live with my pain one more day. For months, my body felt like a huge ghetto blaster with twelve rock stations on at the same time, with the volume as high as it would go. The ghetto blaster would bulge and bloat because it couldn't hold all that sound. I knew that my father had made my "childbody" feel too many intense and conflicting feelings. My body would have to blow up. It couldn't contain all of them.

One day, I began to realize that this is what my "nightchild" felt — the "nightchild" I hated with all my being. All of a sudden I thought, "If I can't make it through one more day at age forty-seven, how did she survive this when she was only seven?" I began to have respect for this ugly, dirty, unlovable, and unacceptable "nightchild" whom I had sentenced to death.

If you are engulfed in body pain, anger, and hopelessness, remember: Recovery is a *process*. You can work through these feelings, but it takes guts. It means looking terror right in the eye.

Please do not minimize your violation by saying, "But I was only fondled," or "It only happened a few times." We are learning that one violation can traumatize a child forever. Whenever you hear yourself starting to say, "But it was only —," STOP. A violation is a violation. Honor your process. If shame is overwhelming for you, as it was for me, stop *acting* ashamed. "I am an incest survivor." SAY THE WORDS. Say the words with pride. We survived with no one to help us. Do not be ashamed of yourself; be ashamed of your violator. I was fifty-three before I stopped feeling ashamed. I stopped feeling ashamed largely because I stopped acting ashamed. Try it.

For those of you who are in pain, I wish I could bring you into the glorious world I now live in. I have such peace, calm, quiet. There were many months when I thought I was losing my mind, when I thought I couldn't hang on one more day, but I assure you, the pain ended. I have peace. Remember during your journey, recovery has an end — I promise — if you do your work. My thoughts are with you. I hold the precious child you were in my heart.

Marilyn Van Derbur
former Miss America and
incest survivor

INTRODUCTION

There is something wonderful about touch, especially for children. After a long day at school, a hug says "Welcome home, sweetheart, I love you!" The squeeze of a hand on the way to the doctor's office can mean "It's all right, I am right here with you." When a rough and tumble game of family football is done, a pat on the back says "You did a good job!"

In today's world, where children grow up so quickly, we need to use touches like these to remind children that they are special, that we love them, care for them, accept, and support them. After all, isn't that what we all want from those around us?

But what about touches that leave a hurtful impression on a child for a long, long time? That is what sexual abuse does. It inflicts invisible scars, sometimes for life. Abuse sows images and ideas that create deeply rooted feelings of anger, distrust, and revulsion.

For a multitude of reasons, our society is unable and unwilling to confront the reality of childhood sexual abuse. Yet sexual abuse is real, and it impairs the lives of hundreds of thousands of children and adults every year. It damages not only the child victim, but the offender, the non-offending parent, and the entire family structure as well. It also affects the adult survivors well past their childhood, as they continue to deal with the day-to-day impact of their childhood trauma.

Another form of severe sexual abuse that professionals are just beginning to recognize is that of ritualized abuse, abuse that is perpetrated against a child in the name of some religion or ideology. Most ritual abuse survivors report that this type of abuse is connected with Satanic worship, but there are many other cults, convictions, and religions that offend our children today.

One of the ways severe sexual abuse impacts some survivors is to cause them to create different personalities within themselves in order to deal with the trauma of their abuse. This is called multiple personality disorder. I have included some powerful writings by multiples that discuss this survival technique.

Sexual abuse also impacts the partners of survivors. I believe that if your partner was sexually abused, you, as a partner, have also felt the effects of sexual abuse in your life. Partners of survivors often face the pain, terror, and fear with the survivor and therefore also begin to experience the post-traumatic symptoms of the abuse.

The purpose of this book is to help you understand and accept the reality of the physical, emotional, and spiritual pain that sexual abuse creates. I want to encourage you to use *Triumph Over Darkness* as a tool in therapy. First, know what your own abuse story is. If you do not have memories of your abuse, you need to explore all possible reasons for your inner pain. Then, identify with the contributors in this book to know that you are not alone in your recovery. You might find some ideas within these pages that will help you to express your own feelings and thoughts. Be assured that this book faces the impact of sexual abuse squarely. I believe that a survivor needs to experience his or her own feelings, deal with the reality of those emotions, and then go on to heal the scars, which many not be visible but are deeply felt.

Bringing the heretofore secret feelings of abuse survivors out of the shadows may also assist therapists, parents, spouses, and all others who really care about and want to stop the continuing effects of abuse. It is my wish that this book play a role in protecting the children of today from experiencing the trauma of abuse. But above all, it is meant to offer support and encouragement to those who have already experienced abuse and are ready to take bold steps out of the darkness and into the light.

Please know that, for most, this will not be an easy book to read. I encourage you to take good care of yourself while working through the chapters. Put on warm slippers as you walk through this work; realize that at times you may also need a soft blanket, a cup of tea, or a hand to hold. Some of the entries may be difficult to integrate. Trust your inner self to pace you on this journey. Sometimes, take off your warm slippers to rest and soak your feet.

The book covers all sides of the recovery process, from the darkness and fear that come from the trauma of the abuse, to the light and hope that is found in recovery. Above all, please know that recovery is possible, and that I believe in the concept of recovery as outlined here, or I would not be working in this field. You can do it! Believe in yourself — I do.

Unfortunately, sexual abuse of our children continues to occur every few minutes, and the recovery of adults still dealing with the trauma must go on. I look forward to the day when a book such as this will be obsolete. Until then, I remain committed to assisting individuals in their personal recovery. Now, I appeal to you to make your personal commitment to see child abuse end in your lifetime.

Finally, it is my desire that *Triumph Over Darkness* will be a resource to guide you through and out of the fear and darkness to discover the beauty that lies within.

A Discussion Of Terms

The following is a list of terms that will appear throughout this book. While these terms may have additional meanings, I have narrowed their definitions to focus specifically on the topic of the book: recovering from the trauma of childhood sexual abuse. Because recovery is intensely personal, I often have my clients create their own definitions for various terms. If any of the following definitions do not fit you and/or your personal experience, rewrite the term in the back of the book with your own definition.

COUNTERTRANSFERENCE: As a result of the therapist's own unresolved issues, she/he develops positive or negative feelings or views about a client, which affects her/his ability to treat that client. I believe that therapists should always be working on their own "issues" in order to stay on top of any possible countertransference. Unresolved countertransference can permanently damage the client-therapist relationship.

DENIAL: Refusing to acknowledge something in your life in an effort to defend yourself against the stress and/or anxiety it might cause you if you confronted it. Denial is acting as though something did not happen, when, in fact, it did.

FLASHBACK: Reexperiencing the trauma and abuse you experienced as a child. Flashbacks usually occur when you have been confronted by some kind of personal trigger. A good test to tell if you are having a flashback is to ask yourself if the emotions you are feeling are too intense for the situation you are in. If the answer is yes, you are probably having a flashback. Flashbacks can take the form of:

VISUAL MEMORIES: in which you may actually see the abuse as it happened to you.

BODY MEMORIES: in which your body feels the abuse that was inflicted upon you as a child. You may have inexplicable bruises as a result of body memories.

AUDITORY MEMORIES: in which a flashback is triggered when you come across a personal trigger such as a familiar sight, sound, smell, taste, or touch. The trigger is then considered an auditory memory.

GROUP THERAPY: A gathering of survivors, either with or without therapists, where people with similar issues come together to work on them. The part of group therapy that is most helpful is the support you receive from other participants.

HYPERDEPENDENCE: An excessive dependence on a therapist or other support person. This dependence allows the survivor to remain immobile and discourages personal growth. Normal dependency occurs in all therapeutic relationships; it is hyperdependence that is toxic. If a patient is unable to go a single day without talking to her/his therapist, is unable to make simple life decisions without the therapist's permission, or is having three- to four-hour therapy sessions daily, she/he is hyperdependent and her/his therapist is failing to empower her/his client, which is essential to personal growth.

INTIMATE PARTNER: Someone who, in addition to being a supporting partner, is sexually intimate with the survivor, such as a lifetime companion or a spouse.

JOURNALING: Writing down your thoughts, feelings, and actions. Journaling is an integral part of the recovery process. It allows you to clarify your feelings and motivations in the moment and provides a record of your progress.

MULTIPLE PERSONALITIES: A defense mechanism to deal with the brutality of childhood abuse. An individual with multiple personalities has divided aspects of her/his personality into separate but complete functioning personality states, known as "alters." Multiples usually experience periods of amnesia when the main or core personality does not know that alters are present and in control of the body and surrounding environment. Alters can range in age from birth to many years older than the actual chronological age of the core personality. Early in treatment, personalities rarely appear simultaneously; they vie for consciousness. In most cases one personality, or alter, is totally unaware of the other(s).

NEGATIVE SPECIALNESS: Dr. John Briere created this term and has a lengthy definition for it. However, for the purposes of this book, I use the term to mean using the negative and painful events in your life to feel unique or special in some negative way. For example: "I am so bad, awful or rotten, that no one could possibly want to be my therapist, so I am not ever going to get well."

POST-TRAUMATIC STRESS: An emotional reaction that occurs anywhere from a few months to many years after the sexual abuse. When a person experiences post-traumatic stress, old coping styles and stress management skills stop working the way they have in the past, and physical or emotional symptoms appear as a result of the trauma.

PRIMARY THERAPIST: The person who provides your individual therapy. She/he should be networking or communicating with the rest of your health care providers (with your signed authorization) to provide you the best possible care.

RECOVERY: Recognizing and reclaiming your abusive past, understanding that it is a part of your life's history and your identity. Recovery includes feeling the loss and grief of the past and finally letting go of the trauma and its effects, which were once an integral part of your survival.

REPRESSION: A defense mechanism that forces painful life events, thoughts, feelings, and ideas into your unconscious. The repressed material may remain active in the unconscious and affect your conscious life.

RITUAL ABUSE: An especially brutal form of abuse that includes sexual, psychological, spiritual, and/or physical abuse. This type of abuse typically coincides with rituals and is usually inflicted on victims by members of a cult in the name of an ideology. Many survivors of abuse identify their abuse as being Satanic in nature; however, there are other ideologies that perpetrate this abuse. Victims range in age from children to adults. In most instances, the abuse occurs over a period of time and is often accompanied by mind control and/or brainwashing.

SELF-CARE: Nurturing yourself during your recovery. For survivors of incest, it is giving yourself the love that you needed from parents and family members but did not receive. Realize that no one can really care for you as well as you can care for yourself.

SEXUAL ABUSE: A sexualized trauma acted out upon a vulnerable or powerless person. The offender is motivated by the sexual and/or emotional satisfaction he/she derives from abusing. Sexual abuse includes one or more of the following:

    COVERT ABUSE: Exploitative behaviors or attitudes such as unsettling looks and/or touching, sexual language, overtones, and/or innuendoes.

    OVERT ABUSE: Fondling, anal, vaginal or oral penetration, rape, exposure to or inclusion in pornography, and/or group exploitation.

    INCEST: When a family member, close family friend, family service provider or caretaker uses their power, resources, and/or knowledge to force a child into sexual activities.

SILVER THREAD: A person you knew when you were a child who was not your abuser and who did not deny your abuse, pain, and trauma. A person who caused you to hold on and not give up on yourself. A silver thread is usually a very special adult who, even if you did not see her/him very often, brought a little light to your darkness. Think back on your life to a pleasant memory and see who is associated with it; she/he is likely to be your silver thread.

SUPPORTING PARTNER: Someone who cares about the survivor and has chosen to be there for support through the thick and thin of personal recovery. Supporting partners might include other survivors, non-offending family members, clergy, a therapist, teachers, or anyone else of your choosing who is nonabusive. The important thing to remember is safety; a safe supporting partner will not foster a hyperdependence in you.

SURVIVOR: Someone who was a victim of abuse but realizes that the victimization is over. She/he has survived the trauma with whatever coping skills she/he could find, and she/he is now working toward rebuilding her/his life and seeking emotional health.

THERAPEUTIC RELATIONSHIP: The relationship between the client and the therapist. Some examples of things that **do not** occur in a healthy therapeutic relationship are socializing with your therapist or anyone in your therapist's social system, having sexual relations with your therapist, providing services in "trade" for therapy (there are other ways to get therapy when funds are limited that do not compromise the therapeutic relationship), working for your therapist, working on a book with your therapist, and having a therapist who is also your teacher.

THRIVER: Someone who has triumphed over the darkness. Someone who has worked through much of her/his sexual abuse history, processed it with applicable feelings and resolution, replaced destructive coping styles with healthy ones, and is able to focus on life in the moment. I believe recovery is possible. It is hard work, but it is possible.

TRANSFERENCE: An important and necessary part of a therapeutic relationship, in which the client unconsciously begins to revive and relive attitudes and behaviors that were present in the parent-child relationship or other significant childhood relationships. In this way, the client can work through unresolved relationships and conflicts by projecting feelings and attitudes onto the therapist, who, in turn, identifies them as they are related to a childhood relationship, thus helping the client to work through the issues in a safe way.

TRIGGERS: Normal life events, like a smell, a sight or a sound, can cause you to suddenly feel as if the abuse is happening right now. Flashbacks will occur, but if you can train yourself to know what your triggers are and how to respond to them, they will be less traumatic for you.

VICTIM: Someone who is currently being sexually, emotionally, and/ or physically abused or has recently experienced such abuse.

Statistics On Sexual Abuse

According to a Congressional Committee Report, 50 to 80 percent of all sexual abuse crimes committed in the United States go unreported.

- One in three females has been sexually assaulted by age nineteen (FBI, Uniform Crime Reports).

- One in seven males has been sexually assaulted by age nineteen (FBI, Uniform Crime Reports).

- Most rape victims are between ten and nineteen years of age. One quarter of rape victims are under the age of twelve (FBI, Uniform Crime Reports).

- 63 percent of incestuous fathers engage in some type of penetration (Williams and Finkelhor, 1992).

- Women who were sexually abused by their mothers usually report violent abuse and object penetration, while men who were abused by their mothers usually report being treated like a lover (Everet, 1987).

- 65 percent of survivors of child abuse suffer from depression (Sedney and Brooks, 1984).

- 34 percent of women sexually abused before age fifteen have a history of eating disorders (Oppenheimer, Palmer and Brandon, 1984).

- 27 percent of survivors have a history of drug or alcohol addiction (Briere, 1984).

- 82 percent of offenders committed their first offense before age thirty (Groth, 1979).

- 90 percent of offenders are male (Finkelhor, 1984).

- 60 percent of all sexual abuse occurs in the home of the victim or the offender (Grossman, 1983).

- 40 percent of all sexual abuse takes place over a period of time ranging from weeks to years (Brownmiller, 1976).

ADULT SURVIVORS
OF SEXUAL ABUSE:
What We Would Like You
To Know About Us

1. We grew up feeling very isolated and vulnerable, a feeling that continues into our adult lives.

2. Our early development has been interrupted by abuse, which either holds us back or pushes us ahead developmentally.

3. Sexual abuse has influenced all parts of our lives. Not dealing with it is like ignoring an open wound. Our communication style, our self-confidence, and our trust levels are affected.

4. Putting thoughts and feelings related to our abuse "on the back burner" does not make them go away. The only way out is to go through these emotions and process them.

5. Our interest in sexual activity will usually decline while we are dealing with this early trauma. This is because:

   • We are working on separating the past from the present.

   • Pleasure and pain can sometimes be experienced simultaneously.

   • It is important for us to be in control, since control is what we lacked as children.

   Sometimes we need a lot of space. Pressuring us to have sex will only increase our tension.

6. We often experience physical discomforts, pains, and disorders that are related to our emotions.

7. We often appear to be extremely strong while we are falling apart inside.

8. There is nothing wrong with us as survivors — something wrong was *done* to us.

9. Sometimes others get impatient with us for not "getting past it" sooner. Remember, we are feeling overwhelmed, and what we need is your patience and support.

- Right now it is very important to concentrate on the past. We are trying to reorganize our whole outlook on the world; this won't happen overnight.

10. Your support is extremely important to us. Remember, we have been trained to hold things in.

   - We have been trained not to tell about the abuses. We did not tell sooner for a variety of reasons: We were fearful about how you would react, what might happen, etc.

   - We have been threatened verbally and/or nonverbally to keep us quiet, and we live with that fear.

11. Feeling sorry for us does not really help because we add your pain to our own.

12. There are many different kinds of people who are offenders. It does not matter that they are charming or attractive or wealthy. Anybody — from any social class or ethnic background, with any level of education — may be an offender. Sexual abuse is repetitive, so be aware of offenders with whom you have contact. Do not let them continue the cycle of abuse with the next generation of children.

13. We might not want or be able to talk with you about our therapy.

14. We are afraid we might push you away with all our emotional reactions.

   You can help by:

   - Listening

   - Reassuring us that you are not leaving

   - Not pressuring us

   - Touching (with permission) in a nonsexual way

15. Our therapy does not break up relationships — it sometimes causes them to change as we change. Therapy often brings issues to the surface that were already present.

16. Grieving is part of our healing process as we say goodbye to parts of ourselves.

EFFECTS OF SEXUAL ABUSE

The following is a list of **some** of the effects survivors experience as a result of sexual abuse. When using this list, check the items that apply to you and add your own. The effects of abuse are not the same for everyone. They depend upon a variety of factors including length and frequency of the abuse, severity and type of abuse, age at which the abuse began, the relationship between the offender and the survivor, and the response of others if the survivor reported the abuse. Use this list to help you realize that you are not alone in your struggle.

- Isolation due to the inability to form healthy, satisfying relationships
- Loneliness
- Self-hatred
- Shame
- Obsessive or compulsive guilt
- Inability to trust
- Fear of having a family
- Difficulty identifying feelings
- Avoidance of people who are the same sex as the offender
- Loss of self-confidence
- Poor self-esteem
- Difficulty with normal sexual responses
- Addiction to drugs, alcohol, food, etc.
- Self-mutilation
- Self-destructive behaviors
- Repetition of cycles of sexual abuse, physical abuse, addiction and other forms of self-harm
- Fear of relationships
- Constant searching for the love and acceptance from others that should have been provided by your family.

- Childlike feelings
- Dissociation and detachment
- Attacks of panic
- Low expectations or fatalistic life view
- Debilitating fear
- Anger towards authority and those in positions of power (as the offender was)
- Poor body image
- Difficulty with personal boundaries
- Identity crisis
- Feeling incomplete due to the separation between your emotional and physical selves
- Nightmares
- Physical illness for which there is no apparent cause
- Unconscious self-sabotage
- Rageaholic tendencies

A COMMITMENT
TO RECOVERY CEREMONY

When you are ready to make your commitment, plan a ceremony. Use candles, music, and/or gifts; invite special people in your life to be present with you. These are the people who will be there through the good times and the hard times. If you don't have anyone like that in your life right now, have the ceremony by yourself. Incorporate the following vows into your ceremony:

For survivors:

I, _____ (survivor's name), do hereby make a commitment to myself and to _____ (add the name of your partner and/or support people) to begin (or continue) my childhood sexual abuse recovery, this the _____ day of _____, 199__. I promise myself to continue working through the effects of my abuse until I reach recovery. I have made the choice to recover because I want to improve the quality of my life, and I realize that the only alternative is to continue in pain and suffering. I create this document as a symbol of my dedication to recovery.

For partners:

I, _____ (add the name of the partner or support people), do hereby make a commitment to myself and to _____ (survivor's name) to assist her/him in her/his childhood sexual abuse recovery, this the _____ day of _____, 199__. I promise you, _____ (survivor's name), that I will stand by you as you continue to work through the effects of abuse in your life. I have made the choice to assist in your recovery because I care about you and want you to improve the quality of your life. I promise to explore my own issues, take care of myself during this process, and work on improving myself. I create this document as a symbol of my dedication to your recovery.

CHAPTER ONE

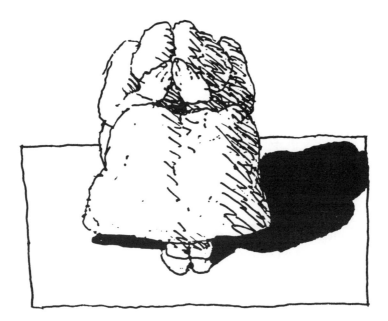

ECHOES FROM
THE DARKNESS

GAMES

She was little. So very little. And small. Inside, too. Her very youngness was a threat. It reminded him that he was getting old. It mocked the dried-outness of his useless life, that freshness of hers. He wanted some of her life, her joy for himself. He wanted to possess it. He wanted to possess her.

It started out innocently enough — on her part. In her trust and adoration she saw nothing strange in them shedding their clothes. She reveled in the freedom from restraint and with hilarity and abandon leaped and giggled just in her own skin.

Over days and weeks and months, the game increased in scope. Touching games escalated into serious business. More and more was required and she found she had to work — to perform — whether it was fun or not. And somewhere in the seventh month it stopped being fun.

The familiar horsie game, the sensuality of flying high, of being the queen of all the land, making her big daddy her slave, developed a subtle twist. The illusion of the control she thought she had was slipping. More and more her Prince Valiant overrode her queenly decisions. More and more the game went on — past her decree to stop.

And then, in that awful seventh month, her decrees became awful, wrenching pleas. The prince became a great, fire-breathing dragon. He breathed into her very being a horridness and vileness that choked her and made her retch but not cry out.

Not yet.

And he laughed. And he reached inside her and pulled out her joy and her trust and her sense of her very self and he ate them up and vomited them all over her cringing, fearful little body. He was enraged that her joy had not become his own, that it refused to stay inside him and he turned on her in a fury which unleashed the devil in him.

He beat her with his fists and when she did not cry out, frozen with fear, he cursed her and shook her and knocked her into walls and furniture.

And with a single cry, a hardly-heard moan, her frozen fear melted into a gray daze of protecting clouds, a thin attempt to stretch over the deep wound in her spirit. And he dropped her on the floor at his feet.

When he walked away from her, the despoiled joy that had once been hers returned in a sinister evil form. It mocked her and tormented her with hissing, vile sounds that made this tightness of her skin a prison out of which she could never escape. Those sounds became her jailers, their monotonous gyrations enveloping her, seducing her, freeing her from peace and enslaving her in their merciless tyranny.

Even though HE walked away. And left her on the floor. They NEVER will. They never will.

Janet W.

A PROGRESS REPORT ON JANET

I am not completely recovered, and I don't know if recovery from something so traumatic and devastating can ever be termed "complete." Certainly the horror of it will never be entirely erased. Yet I am better than I have ever been before. I am continuing to heal hour by hour, day by day, and week by week.

In my case healing is coming by a combination of things including prayer, God's healing and a very wonderful psychologist. I am able to talk about the past traumas, including the feelings associated with them. As I do, I am beginning to be free of them.

The journey isn't over yet, but I can see the light at the end of the tunnel. I no longer consider suicide daily. I no longer hurt myself with razor blades or bruising. I seldom slip into the deep dark despair that used to be my closest companion. I am better, much better, and I thank God for that.

THE RETURN

The horrors return
in the night
in my dreams
in my reality.

The smell
of old booze
and garlic
Your hot breath
smelling up my room
telling me to be quiet
holding me down.

I struggled
you tried to kiss me
slobbering, pungent.
I held my mouth closed tightly
my legs even tighter
gripping my thighs together
my ankles intertwined
Leave me alone.
I'll show you what it's like
Fighting back, scratching.
Then the pillow
Over my face,
I was smothering
I was dying . . .
groping hands
pulling my legs apart
pain, horror,
betrayal . . .
Raped . . . yes daddy, you showed me what it was like.

Pamela J.

A PROGRESS REPORT ON PAMELA

So much has changed in my life. After sending off the writing I put it away, the incest, the memories, the pictures, the feelings, in a tidy little box hidden in the closet. I was so sure I was finished with it and could get on with my life. For the next two years I continued to drink and use drugs to block the feelings and the fears, until I hit bottom. I was an addict and an alcoholic who was tired of running. I placed myself in a very intensive treatment program where I dealt with my alcohol and drug problem and with some of my incest issues. I have continued to remain clean and sober for sixteen months through active participation in a twelve-step program.

For the first time in my thirty-four years on this earth, I am involved in a healthy relationship. This has prompted me to pull out these writings and take a good look at how putting my incest in a box tied up with strings was not the way to heal myself.

I entered therapy again with the same therapist I'd seen years before. Today as a clean and sober woman I can face the fears of my past. I am just beginning to discover Pammy, that little girl who got lost so long ago. She is the key to my reconciliation with myself. I embrace her, forgive her, believe her, and love her.

I've discovered that healing is a process. Before, I wanted an instant cure and sought to alleviate the pain through alcohol and drugs. My healing is ongoing. I've hung up my shoes. Sign me healthy and happy.

LYNN'S STORY

Once upon a time, there was a little girl named Lynn. Lynn had a mythic ancestor named Cody. Cody became Lynn's guide when she was three years old and remained with her all her life.

Cody possessed the wisdom that comes with age and experience. Lynn didn't always realize it, but Cody was always with her. Cody was responsible for helping Lynn to survive life's struggles as best she could.

The first trauma Cody tried to help with involved Lynn's stepfather. He was a mean man who didn't like little girls. Cody gave Lynn courage to tell the truth. Cody never dreamed she would be ignored. It seemed drastic, but Cody was forced to teach Lynn how to survive without having to depend on others. Thankfully, with Cody's help, Lynn was always able to avoid being alone with her stepfather. Unfortunately, Lynn also learned not to trust and not to feel. From that point on, Cody knew it was his duty to find ways to transform Lynn's spirit so that she could truly live and not just survive.

Sadly, Lynn's struggle to survive continued. She was led to a hospital with another mean, abusive man. This time, Cody knew Lynn would need more help than he could give. It was a gift of grace when Cody guided Lynn to Mrs. Banks' writing class. She intuitively knew how to bring out the best in Lynn and keep her safe, for a time at least.

And then, the girl became a woman. Cody's challenges had just begun. For every step forward in becoming the woman God created her to be, there were two steps backwards. Cody never lost faith, even though it appeared that Lynn did on occasion. Cody managed to lead Lynn to other significant people so that no matter how alone she might feel, someone was always there for her. In this way she survived her alcoholism, treatment for cancer and her father's suicide.

Gradually, Cody's job got easier. Lynn seemed more willing to accept his nurturance; and her setbacks became fewer. Cody realized he would probably always have to help Lynn in the process of learning to live, rather than merely survive, but finally, Lynn had come to share that goal. And they all lived happily ever after.

Lynn M.

A SENSE OF INTIMACY

Intimacy looks like a stained glass window in the sunshine.
Intimacy sounds like children laughing on a spring day.
Intimacy feels like holding hands at the movies.
Intimacy smells like baby powder after a bath.
Intimacy tastes like chocolate chip cookies warm from the oven.

Abandonment looks like a broken window pane.
Abandonment sounds like winter wind whistling.
Abandonment feels like a hug that didn't happen.
Abandonment smells like a musty attic.
Abandonment tastes like lukewarm milk.

If all my senses tell me intimacy is better, why am I so afraid?
Will abandonment always offer a sense of safety?
Will you hold my hand and eat chocolate chip cookies with me?

Lynn M.

A PROGRESS REPORT ON LYNN

For the past year and a half, I've been in group or individual therapy for sexual abuse. I am also recovering from an eating disorder and chemical dependency. Although recovery hasn't gotten any easier, I no longer have to constantly question whether or not it's worth it. It is.

Surprise

i said
if i told
my father would never speak to me.
my mother would have a nervous breakdown.
my oldest brothers would have marital problems.
my perpetrator brothers would be exposed and get sick.
their perpetrator friends would deny — and then laugh.
my sister would hate the chaos and gain weight —
all the while denying.
my youngest brothers would not understand —
but they really would
sexual abuse runs in families you know — a filthy epidemic.
society would point their fingers.
i sure do have a lot of power.
the world sure does revolve around me.

well nothing much happened
the world continued to spin on its axis
everyone denied
and
i
got
healthier.

Cecilia

NOT INCEST

My sister cried not incest
My mother cried in rage not incest
I took Xanax and yodeled and my knuckles
went white saying, not incest, not rage
One universal voice said Don't speak
I went tight saying no bad words
Odious, queer thoughts formed in my head till
I went deaf on the great taboo, went blind
and tight and white saying not incest

Sandra Joel A.

HEY YOU

I wrote Hey You on Friday night after work, after first cancel-
ing my plans to go out with a friend, as I felt too depressed and
fatigued to be with anyone. I felt an unexplained sense of impending doom, terrible isolation and confusion as I took off my nurse's
uniform to take a warm bath and to attempt to relax a little. My
sense that something bad was about to happen persisted through
the bath as did the badgering voice inside my head saying . . . why
do you have to be depressed all the time, what's the matter with
you anyway, always thinking of yourself, never thinking of anyone
else, grow up. Words I learned from my mother at a very early age.

I've had enough therapy and have enough health to know that
when I'm feeling this low, it's really important to intervene on my
own behalf, before I sink even lower. My incest group leader had
mentioned in group the night before that I might want to write a
letter to my father, as I had been struggling with a lot of unanswered questions. I knew he had sexually abused me many
times, but could only remember one particular incident clearly. So
I decided to start a note to him this Friday night.

Within one hour my Hey You letter came out through what I
call automatic writing. It isn't truly automatic, but the words pour
out without censorship, and with each word comes an enormous
sense of power. The power I never had as a child becomes mine as
words and fury hit the paper. I write to exhaustion and then read
what is before me. And with the reading and rereading comes a
sense of relief to have so much bad stuff outside of me and to see
this bad stuff for what it really is. Not an ugliness that *is* me, but
a badness that was *done to* me.

This particular piece was healing for me, as I had never before
been able to express any anger at all toward my father. He was a
sick man, he was an alcoholic, he couldn't help it, he suffered so
much throughout his life . . . but my father committed some really
heinous crimes against me and my two siblings and I feel it is important for me to look at them now and work through the pain, so
I can become the best me possible. Perhaps then, any goodness I
might have will counteract his evil.

Hey You!

That's right, I'm talking to you. I won't call you Dad or Father or Daddy or Joe or Joseph. You are nothing more than a Hey You and you don't even deserve that much courtesy. You deserve to be beaten and tortured and humiliated in prison where no one calls you by name, where things are done to you without salutation, where syphilitic homosexuals come up to you from behind. Then thugs, that's right, hey you, big mean fat nasty thugs who use brass knuckles to punch your fat belly so hard and so repeatedly that you double over, cry out in pain. I hate you, Hey You. I hate you. I want you back here on this earth. Death is too good for you. I hate you and I can't find enough bad words to explain you.

You hurt me, nameless. You hurt me more than you were hurt in my imaginative pay-you-back prison. You used me. I was nothing to you but a toy, not even a treasured toy. I was your disposable, breakable ten-cent toy. You bought me for cheap. You used me and disposed of me and repurchased me time and time again. Your dimes came out as fast as the click, click, click of an ice cream man's silver belt-changer. Dimes at the flick of a finger. Dimes to buy JoAnnie, breakable, throw-away baby doll.

Did you know me, nameless? Did you ever wonder who the hell I was? Could you never see the flame of my intelligence behind my provocative child eyes? You seduced me. You stole my innocence. You jobless, worthless, "un-man" — man. I had nothing but abstracts as your child. Abstracts like purity, cleanliness and innocence. You punctured my purity with your blade, leaving me with more abstracts like pain and shame and desperation.

You summoned me with a "let's go" toss of your head. I responded like a co-conspirator, a really small and earnest cooperator. I wanted your love. We'd go someplace together, you remember where, and you would drip my name like honeyed sex juice down your engorged and trembling lip, "Baby doll, come here to Daddy." How dare you call yourself that name! You are a nameless. You are abstract, like the fetid black air seeping from your humid dark grave.

You scared me, nameless. I shake now as I write to you. Where did you take me? Where did we go? What did you do to me? Why do I tremble now? Why am I compelled to write this? Anger has quieted down and in its place is fear. I've been thinking a lot about all the evidence, nameless. My night terrors, calling out, "No, no, no, please help me. I'm going to die," each night in my sleep, in my thirty-ninth year, I cry out to someone, "Oh dear God, please help me." There is too much evidence against you, nameless. Two therapists finding puzzle pieces to fit the rape puzzle, the father-daughter-did-it-together puzzle, the JoAnn-has-blocked-out-terrifying-memories puzzle. You know the answer, nameless. You were there and you were drunk. You hurt me so badly I blacked out. I remember forgetting. Was it the couch, you slippery dick of a man? Your slimy tongue in my mouth, your whale of a body pumping away on me, pressing out my held breath with each clumsy thrust and pump. Each bump and pump pushing me further and further away from consciousness. Each breath out lowering me deeper and deeper into the bloody abyss.

I am remembering.

JoAnn

A PROGRESS REPORT ON JOANN

I am doing much better, especially since I became involved with twelve-step programs at Adult Children of Alcoholics and Al-Anon. Working with my spirituality has also turned my life around. The most important step I have taken towards my recovery is to establish a relationship with my own inner child.

I didn't really believe that little girl still lived within me until I found a survivors' group where it was safe to feel and share the outrage, fear, shame, guilt, and sorrow. In this group we used big bats to beat pillows that symbolized our perpetrators. This allowed me to cry and let out all those feelings which were hurting me, and no one else. The grief process could then begin to take the place of the depression.

Whenever I'm feeling really bad and I don't know why, I write to my inner child, little JoAnn, and she writes back. She knows the truth. She knows what is going on even when this grown-up is confused. She really likes to play. She is still afraid of a lot of things though. When she is afraid, she gets a lot of comfort from me. She didn't get that then, but she can get it now and she deserves it.

An Escape

I feel like there is something I have to write down. It is about music. It is about Neil Diamond. In 1982 I married, and there was horrible stuff, and I ended up in a divorce. I remember I felt so trapped. My husband had taken away my driving privileges so I had to go everywhere with him. I could not use the phone without his permission. We lived in an eight-foot-by-twenty-six-foot trailer with one door and the windows were covered with foil. He kept me locked in and wouldn't let me go outside.

During the day he made me stay in a small office and didn't allow me to talk to anyone except his parents. My life was one beating after another and it kept getting worse. He peed in my mouth and he shaved my pubic hair. When I was pregnant I had to have oral sex with him, until I threw up. One time I got the keys and tried to leave. He ran me off the road with another car.

I felt so trapped. I remember sitting behind the stereo and listening to Swan Lake and Neil Diamond records on the headphones. I'd shut my eyes and pray and dream of the day when I'd escape. In the meantime, even though I couldn't physically be free, my mind would escape when I listened to the music. That is how I kept my sanity. I am enormously thankful for Neil Diamond's soft gentle music because it helped me to cope and gave me the courage to escape a horribly violent world.

P. Finigan

PROSTITUTE'S STORY

It was midnight. The "witching hour," she thought with an unhappy grin. She climbed out of her second story window into the supporting arms of her favorite tree and slid down the trunk. She crept down the street, silently, and stepped into a waiting car.

Her pimp's name was Rene. At least, that's what he said. She didn't believe anything he said. Anymore.

Tonight he was in a good mood. She knew that meant he had found several well-paying fucks for her. She didn't know how much they paid Rene but she knew what it took to put him in a good mood. Money, and lots of it. Rene asked a higher price for her services because she was so young. She was thirteen but only looked eleven, if that. Some men wanted to fuck little kids. She didn't care. She knew she'd get what she wanted some day. Soon, she hoped.

Rene dropped her off at his "place." She let herself in the side door and went up to her room. She knew one of those old degenerates would already be waiting for her. That was Rene's style. Let 'em wait. That way they'll be even happier with what they get. She didn't care. She just did what she was told.

She was right. A tubby sixty-plus old man was sitting in her rocker. He was nervous. She could tell by how he jumped when she came in and he stopped biting his nails so abruptly. Well, it was her job to relax him. She knew how. She'd done it hundreds of times.

She smiled her brightest smile and snuggled in his soft lap. "Rock me, Gramps," she whispered. "I'm scared. The boogie man is after me." She giggled as he cuddled her. She ran her finger around his ear and began licking behind his ear and along his neck. She talked little girl talk and made appropriate responses but her mind, her real self, was far away. Her body moved mechanically, performing as if this were the first time, as if they were discovering something new in their own secret world, but it was a lie. But what the hell, she thought. He's paying for his fantasy, I'll give him what he wants. She performed for him and for the three men who came after him that night.

It was when she was with the last john that she let her mind and body come together. She felt a thrill of hope and excitement. Something about this guy told her that she just might get what she had been waiting for. She crossed her fingers and went for it.

While her words and her body performed their very best for him, she kept herself aware in the same room. That was unusual for her but she didn't want to miss anything in this encounter. It was different, somehow.

For one thing, he was younger than most of her customers. He was just about thirty, a little bit thin on the top. Black, slick hair, brown eyes. Serious, real serious. If she cared she would have appreciated his hard lean body, a change from the old flabby ones she usually got. He was slow about getting to it. He'd touch her a little then stare at her for a long time, then touch her again and then stare again. Touch, stare, touch, stare. If she hadn't had this sense about his being the one to give her what she wanted, she would have been nervous about getting back home before anyone woke up and noticed her absence. But the thrill kept her insides aware and the hope and anticipation made the time spent waiting for his move worthwhile.

Finally, he began to undress her. Slowly. He ran his hands all over her body. Then he began to lick her. She cringed inwardly. She hated the licking more than any other part of doing it, but she made her body move the way he wanted and made the little sounds she knew men paid for. He never said a word and she took his silence as her cue. She put her whole self behind her body into pleasing him. Inside she smiled as he responded to her come-ons, and she prepared herself for the penetration. She felt him grow hard and she exuded a false sense of excitement, pulling at him to come in her. Just as he was about to enter her, he cried out and jumped up. He stared at her wildly and she felt fear mixed with excitement and hope.

As he started towards her again she saw a knife in his hand, and relief mingled with fear. She was going to get what she wanted after all.

She couldn't help being afraid, but she knew it would be over soon. As he cut into her, he called her a whore and a slut, a slimy bitch, a child of the devil, and through her pain she agreed. He was speaking the truth and he was cutting the evil out of her. She had led a wicked life, but she would die purged of the guilt she had carried for the past ten years.

As he stopped ripping and started stabbing she sank gratefully into the darkness that she had been waiting for, that had been calling to her for so long, and she rested in the deep velvet blackness and died (if only for a while).

She finally got what she'd wanted.

Janet W.

WHAT MY FATHER TOLD ME

Always I have done what was asked, the melmac
dishes stacked on rag towels, the slack
of the vacuum cleaner cord wound around my hand,
the laundry hung limp from the line.
There is much to do always, and I do it. The iron
resting in its frame, hot in the shallow pan
of summer as the basins of his hands push
the book I am reading aside.
I do as I am told, hold his penis like the garden
hose, in this bedroom, in that bathroom, over
the toilet or my own stomach. I do
the chores, pull weeds out back, shuffle
through stink bug husks and snail
carcasses, pile dead grass in black bags.
At night his feet are safe on their pads, light
on the wall-to-wall as he takes the hallway
to my room.
His voice, the hiss of lawn sprinklers, wet
hush of sweat beneath his hollows, the mucus
still damp in the corner of my eyes as I wake.
Summer ended. School work didn't suit me.
My fingers unaccustomed to the slimness
of a pen, the delicate touch it takes
to uncoil the mind.
History. A dateline pinned to the wall.
And beneath each president's face, a quotation.
Pictures of buffalo and wheat fields, a wagon train
circled for the night, my hand raised to ask the question,
Where did the children sleep?

Dorianne

ODE TO LIFE

Another day of existing without living, of following the lines and signs that give you the appearance of "normalcy," but I know something is different. Though I can escape into a world of robot movements and demands, I cannot crawl outside myself and lose the pain and trauma that pushes at my ribs and threatens to break me and scatter the pieces on the path to nowhere. I am so busy fighting for sanity, whatever that might be, that I have lost contact with my real emotions. I tell myself not to worry, a day will come when I'll understand. And though I let these words spin through me and settle at my feet, I'm still tiptoeing, refusing to get close to myself, my core. If it's there, then so be it. I don't want to know anymore. I don't want to hear or feel or see or speak. I would welcome sensory incapacitation, a blanking out of everything, maybe even breath. Don't misunderstand me, I have no will to die. However, let it be acknowledged, neither have I the will to live. If tomorrow comes, okay. If not, I shall not mourn it as a loss. Nothing can matter that much anymore.

Anonymous

SLIVERS

Have you ever walked through bark dust barefoot? After gingerly stepping through you pause quickly to inspect the soles of your feet and brush away the visible splinters, then continue on your way. The problem, of course, is that not all of the splinters are apparent and you feel a couple still imbedded in the bottom of your foot. You stop, lean against the fence or side of the house and peer intently at the part of your foot that is bothering you. Although you see nothing, you brush away at that spot and begin walking. Sometimes you get all the slivers; other times one or two stubborn slivers remain. They do not cause so much pain that you cannot go on about your business, but you try to walk in a way to avoid feeling the slivers. If you step down too hard, a small pain signal sends a wince up to your face. Eventually, over the course of hours or days, the bark dust either works its way out of your skin or you get a magnifying glass and tweezers and remove the offending particles.

This is an apt analogy for living with incest memories and scars, with the exception being that the slivers go in deeper, and tweezers and a magnifying glass will not do the job.

Some of my slivers

I realized lately that my long-time habit of holding my tongue in a certain way against my teeth and lower lip when I worried stems from when I was a little girl doing oral sex on my father; I would hold my tongue that way so my bottom lip would not get too bashed up against my teeth.

My husband does not affectionately touch my ear lobes anymore because I told him Dad used to hold on to my ears so that if I gagged on his penis I would not quit doing it.

I still cannot fall asleep at night unless I ball my hands into fists, cross my wrists and double up my fists so the knuckles face each others and tuck my fists tightly under my chin. This way my chest and neck are completely protected and I can grip the blanket at the same time, affording meager protection from midnight fondling.

Eventually the slivers do not hurt as much as they used to, unless I step down too hard on a tender spot. I am aware of some of the tender spots, or wounds, so I strive to avoid them. I do not go to movies about rape or violence against women; I am careful about watching Phil Donahue or Oprah Winfrey lest the subject matter come too close to a painful spot in me. I tend to avoid reading the newspaper because the litany of callous violence makes me cry.

Other wounds are more deeply imprinted

One day while watching a Disney movie with my kids, the movie children looking out the windows of a school bus caused me to begin shivering and shaking; I had to leave the room. I do not know what the connection was, but it was powerful.

I often dream of bathtubs or auto accidents and rooms with cement walls. My dream houses usually have narrow uneven stairs with many twists and turns, and lots of windows. I get the magnifying glass out and poke around the dream images with the tweezers, looking for the connection that might release me from the uneasy feeling that there is something ugly and dark festering there. A memory of a previously forgotten rape at my father's hands, perhaps? Is it worse to know, or not to know?

There was a spirea bush that grew in the front yard by the driveway at our house in Oregon. Remembering that bush makes me feel like crying. I do not know why, but I have a theory: Dad would often take me for a ride with him in the family car (a treat for me because I was the oldest, he said). Once we were safely out in the countryside he would pull over and the episode of abuse would begin. Could it be that the spirea bush was a familiar landmark I used as an indicator that it was "over" for the time, that it was safe for my mind to rejoin my body? Perhaps the spirea bush is the only clear memory I could allow myself from that period.

One of my favorite phrases when I was five or six was "That was enough to choke a horse." Gee, I wonder where that could have come from? The only thing I cannot figure out is, was he referring to the size of his penis, or the size of his ejaculation?

These slivers and a host of others, equally tawdry, blunt and painfully deep, continue to be imbedded in my tender skin. My father can never undo what he did to me, to my sister, his sisters, neighbors, and God knows who else. I cringe when I think of the splinters they must carry with them.

In the end the bark dust splinters will work themselves out. The tweezers will rest in the medicine cupboard until next time. My husband will continue to love and support me in my struggle. He knows the slivers are there too.

Vicki P.

A PROGRESS REPORT ON VICKI

I now have ninety-six days clean and sober! I am trying not to substitute food (an old friend) for drugs. Moderate success so far. I try to concentrate on the good things I have: my school work, my family, my group, my cats. I want to like myself better. It comes day by day. The women I get together with on Thursday nights are very special to me, and I give them my deepest thanks.

SURFACING MEMORIES

It is Sunday evening. That is just a reference point of time. I do not think I am aware of the time or day, really. I am fascinated with the way that the blood bubbles up in a little round ball before it breaks its bond and runs downward. I then begin to make criss-cross marks on my lower abdomen and inner thighs. I do not feel a thing. It is just as if I am an observer watching someone else performing this act. I lie awake all night, after taking my sleeping pills, in a state of anxiety. It is a very long, restless night.

Monday — at work. I am feeling anxious and distracted, finding it difficult to hold myself together. In session with Anne I tell her about the self-destruction and dissociation, still feeling the humiliation of having to tell anyone about that aspect of me. I begin feeling more anxious and agitated, wanting to go home. She calmly points out that this whole process usually precedes a memory surfacing. Why didn't I remember that? I usually have a sense of when a new memory is about to show itself and this does not feel like that. But I guess her just saying that was all that was needed.

I am obsessed with my hands, examining them, seeing and feeling slimy, sticky stuff all over them. Dissociated again. She asks if I am hallucinating. Of course not! It is really there! Can't she feel and see it? Then the image of my father rubbing his erect penis around my body and sticky, white stuff squirting out. I try to rub it off and it smears on my hands and I rub it into my eye.

So much fear, pain and shame. The shame is unbearable. Just like the shame of seeing the blood on the tissues when I was injuring myself last night.

Do these memories ever stop?

Nancy M.

YOU KNEW!

You saw and turned away. YOU KNEW!
I write to you now, to tell you that I KNOW.
You say you know nothing about it.
I must be crazy.
I'm crazy?
You were the adult.
You must have known the truth.
I was just a silly kid.

Maybe I do know the truth.
Maybe you don't want to.
Just maybe I am not crazy.
I get to deal with all the feelings.
You get to use your booze
so you don't feel
Just maybe I'm not crazy
Maybe I'm just feeling.

Nancy M.

A PROGRESS REPORT ON NANCY

Some of my writing has come out of a writing group I am currently involved in. I feel this group and the leader's affirmative approach to a subject that is so terribly difficult to express, is the most healing thing that I am doing for myself at this point in time.

Name The Thing

It's a Monster.
> It comes without warning.
> It never goes away.

It's a Monster.
> It attacks children.
> It devours them.

It's a Monster.
> It causes shame.
> It causes pain.

It's a Monster.
> It causes mental anguish.
> It causes torment.

It's a Monster.
> It sometimes creates other monsters.
> So the horrible "chain" continues.

It's a Monster.
> It's name is Sexual Abuse.
> It's name is _____.
>   (your abuser)

Nadine

RECOVERY JOURNEY

The recovery journey is aptly named.
For truly it is a journey
That takes you many places you never otherwise would see.
When you become flat, heavy and low
You sink deeper and deeper
Into the mire of brown muck.
You taste the greenness of the slime
Even as you are blinded with the brown stuff.
Another day you find yourself floating
Miles above the earth
Completely detached
You look way, way down at the world
And can barely make out
The tiny insignificant people
In your life.
And then one time,
You find yourself growing huge
Stretching and inflating
With the awful overwhelming emotion.
And you are very afraid
That unable to contain it all
You will burst.
And one day you shrink
Grow tinier and tinier
Until you can crawl down in the
Corner under the covers of your bed
And disappear.
There is another time
When things go well
And you manage to comfort the
Little girl inside of you

Then you visit the mossy bed
Of the river bank
And watch the soothing blue water
Gently flow past
And you are calm.
Which gives you energy
To enter the spooky black cave
Where you wander blinded by the dark
Knowing evil memories lurk
To take you by surprise
And that the only way to conquer them
Is to let them attack
And through it all you know
That someday
You will spread your wings and soar
Up in the luscious eternity of blue
And you will be recovered.

Mollie

A PROGRESS REPORT ON MOLLIE

I am at the beginning of what looks like a long recovery journey. But I feel that in the few months of therapy I have developed skills and tools that will make the journey possible. I feel stronger and more hopeful than I have ever felt. Through writing I am able to express feelings I do not even realize I have.

LEARNING TO WRITE

A writing class you say?
    Wait a minute, that is not for me.
        I don't write,
            I can't write.
    Well, maybe a case study, an assessment, or evaluations for
work. But to write about myself, I freeze.
    My heart starts racing.
        My stomach ties in knots.
        Yet I endure,
Ending with words,
    Phrases at best.
    Struggling to pull it all together.
        To get my words to flow,
    To express the depth I feel inside.
Feelings of frustration, anger and hurt well up in me, and I
choke.

My fondest childhood memory is searching for discarded pencils in my grandfather's big wicker trash basket. I prized these newly found items and loved to write on old pieces of paper. I was quick to learn that an older pen would often write again if the tip was held to a lighted match. But that was another house. At home, we were not allowed to talk, to laugh, or even to breathe too loud. Lack of opportunity, and torturous threats of death and pain were heavy in the air. There was no paper at home. He said we were not worth the space we occupied or even the space we would use up on paper.

Words and anger confuse me. Words were the messengers for lies — chronic ugly terrible lies that were to become my secrets and even my truth, at times. As a very small child I remember feeling torn between words I heard and how my body and soul responded to those words. I still hear the words ringing in my head today. My dad's voice saying, "If you were not so beautiful I would not have to do this. Besides nothing is happening" and "No one will love you as much as I do. You are lucky I let you live. If you tell, I will kill you."

I remember his gray wrinkled skin with his jutting jaw within an inch from my face, the clutching grip as he squeezed my skin, and most important the black gun. In the same sentence his words would tell me, over and over, that it was all my fault and he was not doing anything. For years I clung to those words. The words that made me wrong, ugly, the "cunt," the filthy one. He spit on me and told me I was nothing. He owned me.

As an adolescent, my own written words caused me pain. After one of his frequent torture sessions, I broke down and wrote that my dad was a bastard and drank too much. I immediately ripped the writing into tiny pieces and scattered the pieces into the big trash can outside. He had searched through the trash, and pieced my words together. His violent eruptions told me loud and clear it was not safe to write, to tell, or to trust my perceptions. My mom's words, her empty promises, ripped right through my heart. I have always known my mom wanted me away, far away and not to need her for anything. Caught in a desperate desire to please the nuns, I felt pushed into asking my mom for help when learning to print my name and later to write my first sentence. I was met with ridicule and humiliation. She would yell, "Just write! What is wrong with you? Just do it alone." As with everything else, I did learn to do it alone. My mom responded to my tears by laughing at me. She continually found delight in my pain and suffering. I wished I could disappear and fade away. On several occasions she spilled coffee or dropped her cigarette on my newly completed homework. Another one of her famous "accidents," I suppose. Here I sit, pen in hand, struggling for the correct grammar, the proper order, stumbling, trying to get my words to flow. I am angry at words, words that lie. I do not trust words. What if I am wrong and nothing happened. Still, within me is a trembling place, frightened, that somehow once again he will search till he discovers my written words and this time he will truly kill me.

For telling.

L.W.

NOT INCEST

"INCEST"
Said the little girl
"NOT INCEST"
Said her mother
"Not incest"
Said her father
"Not incest"
Said her grandma and grandpa
"Not incest"
Said her teachers, preachers and peers
"NOT INCEST"
Cried the little girl

"Disrespectful"
Said her mother
"Withdrawn"
Said her father
"Strong-willed"
Said her grandma and grandpa
"Problem child"
Said her teachers, preachers and peers
"incest"
Whispered the little girl

Julie

PATTY CAKE

Where is my Patty Cake?
Where does she play?
I've been so lonely since she went away.

The laughter is gone
Replaced by cold tears
She does not return for many long years.

Mud pies and castles
We made side by side
Only to crumble when Patty Cake died.

I tried to rebuild them
Alone in my heart
But they resist reconstruction when we are apart.

I call her and plead
Please come share your sweet smile
Let's play together for just a short while.

But she does not hear me
From her land of pain
Though I invite her again and again.

P. Feller

DON'T LET GO

I used to remember falling . . .
I used to remember walking . . .
I used to remember floating among clouds . . .

Now I remember the kisses . . .
Now I remember his eyes . . .
Now I remember the darkness . . .

I cannot stop the pain . . .
I cannot stop the agony . . .
I cannot stop the crying
of the lonely child within . . .

I hold fast to the good memories
I struggle to free the bad.

But how do you free
what you cannot remember?
Remembering is letting go.

Heal yourself slowly . . .
The HEALING will come . . .
The child that cries within you
needs your hand to hold.
So now you are grown on the outside,
but what about within?
Hold that child who is so strong
And both of you can heal together . . .

Don't let go . . .

D. Broussard

A PROGRESS REPORT ON D. BROUSSARD

I was an emotionally, physically, and sexually abused child. I got into a relationship at a very young age that followed the pattern of my childhood and I became pregnant at the age of seventeen. About six years ago I sought help through the local rape crisis hotline where I received the telephone number of a female psychologist.

Over the years I would visit her, slowly discovering through painful flashbacks and lonely times just how severe my abuse was and how dramatically it had affected my life. I am now twenty-eight years old and I see my therapist every week. It has been a very difficult journey just to discover that I have a child within. My counselor has become one of the most important people in my life and even though I still do not trust her completely, I know where the distrust stems from and I am learning to understand my own feelings and thoughts. Slowly, I am learning to trust her more and as the trust grows my healing increases.

Counseling is a difficult and often lonely road to travel, but I have learned so much about myself. Most important, I have learned that I am not crazy and that I will be OK. It has never comforted me knowing that I am not alone, for I do not wish this unending, agonizing pain on anyone. What has been a comfort to me is knowing that there is someone who understands the concepts and the many steps of the healing process. I appreciate your time and consideration for my poem. I would like to be able to assist others in their healing process. The pain never leaves, but it can be handled with help. No one should ever have to deal with the atrocities of childhood abuse alone. Childhood abuse does not make one "crazy."

ECHOES FROM THE DARKNESS:
Insights And Perceptions

After reading this chapter, you may be alarmed by the rawness of your emotions. Some of these feelings may be new, while others are resurfacing after having been put to rest for many years. At this moment you may feel that you would rather not reexperience or deal with this pain. But facing your experiences can get you started on your journey toward wholeness — a journey that simply has no shortcuts.

What can you do when the pain is extreme? During the time you were abused, escape may have been the only way to live. Today you may be using your escape defense mechanism to run away from life, rather than to run toward healing. Escaping is not living, it is merely existing. What was intended to protect you as a child is destructive in your adult life. Realize that you cannot escape from what happened to you or from your feelings. To move toward recovery, you need to face and accept all you have suffered. It might help to explore the ways you escape to discover what you are running from. Depression, suicidal thoughts and/or actions, withdrawing from people, and addictions are some common ways to escape. Remember, there is more to life than merely existing!

Dealing with intense emotions and experiences often weighs survivors down with a sense of hopelessness. It is okay to feel the despair and pain, because what happened to you was NOT okay in any way, shape, or form. It was NOT your fault. Let yourself feel the pain, fear, anger, and any other emotions that arise. Your feelings are valid. Accept them for what they are.

The recovery journey is a lifelong adventure but it does not have to happen in the dark. Find a therapist to walk with you, who will shine a light on the recovery path ahead of you, who will walk with you and not in front of or behind you. You do not have to do this alone.

Perhaps it would help to share your feelings with a safe support partner who is able to listen. Writing, shredding paper, drawing, making a collage of your feelings may also help release some of the intensity. Whatever you do, before you start anything, be sure that you are as safe as you can possibly be. Listen to your inner self and respond as a friend. Accept yourself and the methods you used to survive.

Wendy Ann Wood

CHAPTER TWO

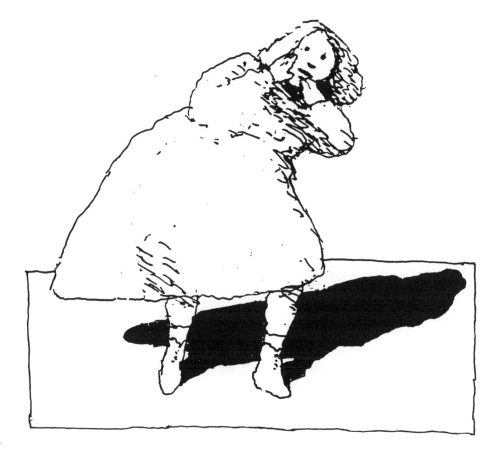

SEEING THE DARKNESS
BEFORE THE LIGHT

TANGLED SCARS

For many years I wondered what was wrong with me. I was paranoid. I had no friends. I didn't like myself. Then I wondered if it was because I was molested as a child. That was just the beginning.

I got married and pregnant at age eighteen. Everything was fine at first, but after the honeymoon was over our problems began. I couldn't make love to my husband because he had brown eyes like my abuser. After a year of arguments and guilt, I decided to seek counseling. After three counselors, I found one who started opening closets for me. I learned that my abuse started at age six months, not to mention losing my virginity at age seven years.

As my memories continued, I became suicidal. The memories got worse, more often. I couldn't cope. I wanted to end the memories so badly, the only way out I saw was to end my life. With the help of my support persons I got past that point. I learned what to do when a new memory arose. When I got a headache or felt tired, I was watchful. Then, when my mind felt like it was spinning tight, I started writing my thoughts. When an embedded memory came to me, I talked it out. For a long period I never wanted to talk or write again, but I learned that was part of the healing process. There was so much inside I needed to express. Through that I found my own identity, instead of continuing to live with my abuser inside of me.

The feelings from being molested are so many, so confusing.

At age nineteen I told my mother what her brutal brother did to me. The support and relief was better than I expected at first. Soon I felt guilty for telling. I felt as though I threw everything on her shoulders. Then, I felt guilty for the guilt she felt. The tension between us grew heavy. I felt as though nothing would ever go back to normal. I was mad at myself for telling. I felt as though I ruined her life. Then I learned she told other family members. I felt like I was stripped of every shield I had. As a secret it had more power, I felt, for if I let the secret out, I knew I could shatter and destroy every vision of a normal family.

Well, shatter I did, but they wouldn't let me destroy their incarnated vision. Not one word was said to me. In a way it was still a secret, except this time it was different. It left a dark cloud lingering, while my scars of pain are still hidden inside. To me they run around like a bunch of hungry ants, blinded by their own darkness. They may never know what went on for those thirteen years, but the strength it took me to survive those years is more than I can say.

The positive side of my incest was that it helped me to help my daughter when she was molested by another sick-minded animal at age two. But that story I will leave for her to tell . . . .

Today I know I can live without my family. I don't need or want anything from them, as I did when I was a child. When they want me they know where I am. If they want my story I will share it. Today I know who I am. I am a twenty-one-year-old woman and I feel good about myself!

My love goes out to any victim of abuse. I only know that it does get better. The tangled cobwebs can be cleaned. Self-esteem can grow so bright! My thanks goes out to every support person who stands behind a victim (especially my counselor and my husband). Each of our lives can become peaceful. We can all find our own identity, and most of all, we can all be survivors!

Beth L.

LOOKING BACK
FIFTY-EIGHT YEARS

My psychiatrist had told me, repeatedly, he was certain I had been raped because of my distrust and fear of men.

One night after retiring, I thought, "If he is right, why can't I remember? I will look in the corners of my memory slowly and carefully." As I relaxed to sleep, horrible sounds came to my mind. Groans, growlings, mumblings, squeals, lips smacking, all incoherent. I sat bolt upright, a gross fear caused my heart to pound wildly and a cold sweat to erupt on my body. I feared for my sanity.

This experience broke the seal on my memory and it all came rolling out. There seemed no way to stop it. I felt as though I were hanging by a gossamer thread to my sanity, and the slightest "bump" would tip me into lunacy. I clung to this thread for two years.

On a spring day when I was nearly five years old, I wandered to an old vacant house one-half block from home. The cellar doors were open and, curious, I went in to inspect the leavings of the last tenant.

A sound of some sort, and my own apprehension made me look up toward the light in the doorway. I saw a man's legs spread wide blocking the way. He came towards me very quickly. "Get in the corner, you brat, and keep your mouth shut." Then he hit me in the head with his fist. My heavy brown knee socks were stuffed in my mouth, obstructing my air passage and causing me to lose consciousness, which was a merciful thing in view of the beating and raping that transpired.

My dad came home after dark, saw the light on in that cellar and came to look for me. I saw those rapist's legs go up those seven steps, only touching them once.

I had a brief moment of consciousness when they put my body in a tub of warm water and cut my dress with scissors. I saw the water was muddy blood.

This rape of their tiny daughter disgraced and frightened my parents. I was not allowed to work through my trauma, but repressed it. It haunted my dreams and affected my emotional life for fifty-five years. Nightmares were always the same: I could not breathe. I would wake yelling and screaming, running from a man I could not see, into a cellar where there was no way out.

Because of repressing this rape-beating, I have felt powerless, afraid of everything and everyone. I was unable to develop to my potential. I will always have emotional scars from my experience. My doors are always locked at home, my car is always locked when I am in it, and when my husband is away I am apprehensive.

They never even looked for my rapist, he was never brought to justice, he is free yet. Who knows how many more victims he has had?

Anonymous

A PROGRESS REPORT ON THIS AUTHOR

I saw a psychiatrist who listened to the horror I had experienced, over and over. It is very important for someone to hear you. I dumped it all on my therapist.

I have stayed away from the house and around people of my age. Walked miles in all sorts of weather — nature has such healing qualities. I have hung on. Telling myself, "I am a special person for my experience."

The worst thing has been that my husband has refused to hear any of it, wants me to forget it.

SEVERING THE IDEALIZED FAMILY

Severing the idealized family from the real family is like severing me into many pieces. Their love, however crazy and painful, is the only love there is, the only love I know. Now I'm supposed to survive the real world without anything. I am lonely to the core. What is going to happen when there is nothing? Is not the craziness and the pain better than nothing at all?

My brain, insides, and life are crumbling at my feet, and nothing seems to be able to hold it all together. I am beginning to feel like a four-year-old orphan who is standing out in the rainy street crying, "Is there nothing else, is this all there is?" I realize this is the martyr thinking, but let's face it, that is the way I feel right now. There is a four-year-old brain living in a thirty-three-year-old person.

I have been asking myself where I go from here. Now that all the dreams are being chipped away, bone raw reality is all that lies before me. I am unable to live in my fantasy world any longer. Feeling stripped of all escapes and so very, very, scared of the road ahead. Somehow, reality is much more frightening than the dreams I used to live with. Scared of myself and my emotion, not knowing who or what to trust, and questioning whether I can even trust myself. Help me! The smell of dead rotting fantasies lingers in my mind, making it hard to forget what has gone before, while scaring up visions of the pain to come.

Anonymous

LETTER UNMAILED

My Dear Friend,

You asked, "Why would anyone want to be touched?"
Your question haunts me
and knowing (recognizing) the underlying question
"How can you forget 'the touch'?"
prompts an answer.

I am blessed that only the "Statue Girl" was touched.
She is the only one who truly remembers
the incidents of my childhood —
and I put her to sleep years ago.
Occasionally she wakes
and to put her at ease
I list my "thank yous" to God.
I touch my husband;
stroke his warm, fuzzy body
and thank God for his presence in my life.
I was alone
isolated,
afraid to venture from my self-sealed walls
and he has listened gently
and (as much as a male can),
has understood.
He remembers and tries to picture
the terror of a young girl
afraid to go to the bathroom
for fear of being cornered and fondled.
I touch him as we make love,
consciously thanking God for his love,
for his ability to assume responsibility
for my fatherless children.
I thank God for blessing me with a man
who is willing to do housework
so I can pursue any one of my compulsive hobbies.
I stroke his arms
and thank God that the arms were there
to hold and comfort me.

I brush his cheek
and thank God that he always turns it
when I am offensive to him.

I rub his shoulders,
loving the closeness that I feel
and thank God that I am able to enjoy that;
Finally, my friend . . .'

I pray.
"Dear Lord, let me forget the past right now and focus all my
energies on this man who has done so much to help me grow. Help
me enjoy the other kind of touch."

Rebecca B.

A PROGRESS REPORT ON REBECCA

The once "impending cloud of doom" that seemed to hang over
my life is gone now. I have worked hard to make it go away. I've
involved myself and my family (including my very supportive husband, Keith) in many different therapy processes. I've seen my
therapists and have been in several group therapy processes. Keith
also went to a group for several months that was for husbands of
abuse victims. He gained much understanding and could see how
"we" relate to many of life's experiences in similar ways.

My journey/struggle is not over — it may never be over. Nearly
every day, I face a paranoia that I need to work out. I fight insecurity
and fear of success and the spotlight success brings. But I can look
at my list of things that I have overcome and I am encouraged.

Today I teach first grade and share a personal safety curricu-
lum with my students. I am pleased that I can tell my children to
say *no*. I am currently working on my own book, which is a Christian testimony of how God's plan has worked for me and how He
can work for others.

My Feelings

I scream!
I scream loud!
Is this the reason no one likes me?
I scream with hate, anger, and love.
Sometimes all mixed up.
But sometimes I just scream
To let my feelings out.
I scream with confusion
I scream with fright
I cry for no reason at all.
Everything builds up in me.
So I just SCREAM.
And we let it build up again.
So I Scream, Scream, SCREAM.

Jody
Age 11

I TOLD MY MOTHER

I told my mother I was molested:
She said I lied.
My face turned black and
My hands beat against my own walls forever.

I told my mother I was molested:
She laughed.
I became a whore and
Searched for a man who could laugh like my mother.
I told my mother I was molested:
She turned her head to the wall and wept large green tears.
My arms fell off to the ground
My private parts withered to scabby bits
My mouth dried up and shut
The earth spun 'round and 'round
And didn't stop once.
I told my mother I was molested:
She kept on making dinner and asked me to make the salad
And set the table.
I set the large black knife at her place.
I put poison in the salad dressing.
I folded a threat in her napkin.
I ran away from home without leaving
And never came back.
I told my mother I was molested:
She fainted dead away.
My eyes rolled back and I saw a snuff movie.
I was the star, I was the audience.
I was the end.

Patty

A PROGRESS REPORT ON PATTY

RECOVERY: I am beginning to know this world after three years of intensive therapy, exclusively devoting my time, minute by minute, and all my thoughts each day towards understanding eighteen years of a traumatic childhood.

The process of healing is to re-cover the wounds in a new way. The bandages of trust and safe closeness have to be woven before they bring solace. I was screaming for help and having to reconstruct myself and weave the bandages all at once.

My therapist and my husband understood that abandonment was my greatest terror. They were patient and constant companions, although it was hard for me to acknowledge or even feel that at the time. Those touches evoked all the remembered disappointments, abandonments and betrayals more strongly than the initial telling of the secrets. It seems every step of healing involves another layer of pain. I protest, I rage, but there is no other way. I refuse to choose death and let "them" win.

Now, three years later, I am covering the wounds and this recovering is done, oh, so differently than the hiding. There are horrendous scars, and things I know I can never do. Sometimes, when I am feeling pretty good, I get a glimpse of those scars and howl with unbearable anguish at what was done to me by my family. I howl, knowing I carry these scars forever.

RECOVERY: learning everyday for the rest of my life how to walk gracefully while carrying a heavy awkward package that has been sutured to my body.

A Symbolic Act

Thrusts of anger into the faceless body
clears the soul of oppressive rage.
The knife's downward path hits its mark
again and again and again.

It is only a survivor's drawing on paper
but it is the face of a prior reality. ·
Free the brain of fury and wrath—
the rampaging storm subsides into grief.

Sobbing sounds and screams fill the air
as forty years of emotions are released.
I am alive and I am powerful.
Killing him in absentia gives me strength.

Paula M.

A PROGRESS REPORT ON PAULA

For forty years I had been able to say that I was an incest victim. It was a passionless, intellectual statement with all emotions
held in check. It wasn't until I began therapy less than two years
ago that I uncovered molestation by a nonfamily member living in
our home. I was not quite five. I am learning to deal with the rape,
sadness, grief, and terror. I am learning how to cry, how to be
angry, how to laugh. Since life is always evolving, I expect one day
to have a serene, happy life.

THIS IS A POEM ABOUT INCEST

The jump-rope girls chant:
"Ice Cream Soda, Delaware Punch,
Tell me the initials of my honey bunch,
A-B-C-D-E-F-G"

G.

Grandpa.

Hide your face, hide your tears
Hide them both for years and years and years

The child is three.
She has one body. She lives there all the time.

Not just sometimes.

I have half a dozen,
one I use for making love, one that cooks breakfast, one
that plays with the kids, one who sits up way too far in the night
worrying about God knows what.

The child is four, the child is fear
the child wears a velvet dress
blood red velvet.
She sits on the fence and smiles at me until I
come to her and pick her up and take
her home.

Nonnie

A PROGRESS REPORT ON NONNIE

I am thirty-six years old. I first remembered the abuse a year ago, after being clean and dry for two years. I have a lot of trouble telling my fantasies from my memories. Some days are better than others. Sometimes I get a flash, like a face seen when a match flares in the dark. I feel unquiet at first, then anxious, then creeping and crippled. I take the day off and let my hands shake all they want to. (What are my hands trying to tell me? What have they done?) Other days, most days, I am fine. I laugh, I play ping-pong, I walk with my young daughter and my dog along the foggy river that runs by my door. I talk to my husband for hours. I can feel the ground under my feet. I'm OK as long as I don't pretend this didn't happen.

PEOPLE DO NOT REALLY WANT TO KNOW

People do not really want to know.
They listen to the news, or
See a show on child molestation
Sigh and say, "That is too bad" or "Poor Kids."
They do not want to know that it could be
Their kid at home in bed molested by a friend or family member
With their life shattered.
People do not really want to have their personal lives
Inconvenienced in any way
Certainly not in the name of safety for another.

People do not really want to know
The child next door is being thrown around the room
Torn from limb to limb
Tattered, battered, shattered
Not to mention loss of self-esteem.

And so they pretend it is not really so
And no one steps in
No one helps the child
Who later becomes an adult
Still struggling, still suffering alone.

For the most part, people still do not want to know what happened
Or allow the feelings that are usually kept locked inside.
People still do not want to know.
Maybe if they really looked
It would hit too close to home.

Lynn

LITTLE ONE

It hurt to be so small
    And have her for a mom
      And need a little help
        To tie my shoe
        To print my name
      Or learn a prayer for school.
She was never nice to me.
No one was.

Lynn

A PROGRESS REPORT ON LYNN

I am a member of a writing group for survivors of sexual abuse. We meet weekly. It is not therapy, yet a safe place to write and share our stories. I work with children who are physically handicapped, emotionally handicapped, developmentally delayed, abused children, drug addicted children and children who are dying. I am active and a firm believer in animal rights as well as children's — those most vulnerable to abuse.

IF NOT FOR GROUP

If not for group,
Where would we be?
Suffering our pain alone,
And oh, so silently.
If not for group,
Who would listen to our fears?
Who would pass the tissue,
For our ever-flowing tears?
If not for group, How could we cope?
Who would lessen our anger,
And give us new hope?
If not for group,
How would we know
That all life's experiences,
Help us all to grow.
If not for group,
How would we learn to be forgiving?
And yes, dear friends,
Our lives are worth living.
Our ever-changing lives,
Are entwined in a loop.
So where would we be,
If not for group?

Liz S.

NASTY WORDS

Slut.
Cunt.
Bitch.
Whore.

Nasty words
many of us learned
in the comfort
of close friends
as jokes,
or idle conversations.

The less fortunate
like me,
learned of them
while being
touched,
slapped,
kicked,
and raped.

Many of us
will forget these words
as time goes by,
but I will not.
I can never forget.

Julie C.

A PROGRESS REPORT ON JULIE

I am happier than I have ever been. I am in school now and am working towards a degree. Since I began talking about my abuse and telling, things have changed a lot. Most of all I began to grow and will continue to. I am still actively working on my recovery and am in a support group. For the first time in my life I am learning to have friends and be supported. I have found out who my real family is, and also who my real friends are. I still have a long way, and do not know if it is ever possible to "recover," but I know I am recovering bit by bit.

I TOLD GOD I WAS ANGRY

I told God I was angry.
I thought He'd be surprised.
I thought I'd kept hostility
quite cleverly disguised.

I told the Lord I hate Him.
I told Him that I hurt.
I told Him that He isn't fair,
He's treated me like dirt.

I told God I was angry.
but I'm the one surprised.
"What I've known all along," He said,
"you've finally realized."

"At last you have admitted
what's really in your heart.
Dishonesty, not anger,
was keeping us apart."

"Even when you hate Me
I don't stop loving you.
Before you can receive that love
you must confess what's true."

"In telling me the anger
you genuinely feel,
it loses power over you,
permitting you to heal."

I told God I was sorry
and He's forgiven me.
The truth that I was angry
has finally set me free.

Jessica S.

A PROGRESS REPORT ON JESSICA

I was in therapy for years, off and on, working on one incident of incest and five other molestations. From my experience, I wrote two booklets for other counselees and their spouses, "What am I doing here?" and "What's gotten into her?"

THE OTHER SIDE OF ME

All my life I have been searching for someone who would make me feel whole. Someone who I could share every bit of my life with no matter how bad it might seem to me. Someone who would understand and not condemn or just be a "yes" man. You know, someone secure enough within himself to accept me for me and yet also be able to accept what might take place with me. I used to believe there was someone who could do this. It has taken me a long time to realize that the person I have been looking for all these years was me. How could I have expected anyone else to accept me for me, faults and all, when I could not do it for myself.

I had been denying myself the one person who would love me no matter what. I never told this person "I love you" and that makes me feel ashamed because I never said "I care about you." But I do! This person is my best friend and sometimes my worst enemy. But she knows me and why I do the things I do. This person is so special and I am real glad that I have finally acknowledged this person. You know the person I am writing about is "me." Strong, levelheaded, assertive and able to cope with anything.

She has kept me from hurting myself, as well as from hurting other people in my life. She is always there and even when I do not want her to, she eventually will help me to be realistic about the hurtful events in my life. She has kept certain events from surfacing until such a time as she knew I would be able to handle it. With every new memory the fear does not take over. Instead I pick my feelings apart so I know exactly how I feel and felt about the abuse.

When I was growing up she was there in my subconscious mind only coming out to rescue me when I needed her. But now I feel her presence all the time. No longer does she hide from me. I feel as though she is blending in with me so that I have a strong but realistic personality. A friend of mine told me a while back that she never knew anyone as "strong or capable" as I am. I did not know then what she meant, but I do now! When a person takes the time to look at herself, as close friends do, it can sure be a shocker.

With each day that passes I learn more about me and why I am the way I am. Life is so wonderful, so full of good and loving people. Sometimes I feel as though I just woke up from a very long sleep, a nightmare full of pain, anguish, uncertainty and failure. Some of the changes in me are unbelievable, but I see and feel them so I know it is real.

Helen M.

A PROGRESS REPORT ON HELEN

I am still in therapy once a week. With each session I am becoming a little stronger and more self-confident. I hope that my article will help someone else realize they are not alone and they are worthy of self-love.

REMEMBERING — NOT REMEMBERING

I go 'round and 'round. Remembering is important — remembering is not important. Will I remember any more? I want to — I don't want to. Not remembering feels bad. Not remembering feels like something is dammed up inside of me — something that wants to come out. I might be frightened. I might be horrified. The not-knowing is a special kind of stress — pressure — that only a few people must know.

A couple of weeks ago I almost fell apart from remembering — not remembering. I had a dream — it was crystal clear. It was a forgotten piece of my history. I woke up thinking, "Yes! That happened. It really happened." It was a moment of clarity and illumination. When I awoke again in the morning it was gone. It had been there and it was gone. I was upset, tearful. I went to church feeling rather odd — pulled into myself. Then that evening I picked a fight with my husband and I blew. I was absolutely full of rage and fury.

I crawled into bed with my rage and was afraid to move. I knew if I got up I would hurt myself. I was trying not to. My husband, once he cooled down and realized that this fight had nothing to do with the topic of the fight and everything to do with the previous night's dream, suggested I call my therapist at home — on a Sunday night. I tried to but only got an answering machine. But I did get in to see him the next day. It was very fortunate as my suicidal feelings were at an all-time high. Over the course of a couple weeks I was able to deal better with my feelings and my vulnerability but the memory was still lost.

And then again I had a memory. This really took me by surprise. My format up until then had been that my memories came back in dreams. But here I was at work, busy but relaxed, my mind just skimming along on a number of topics and a memory just flew in, unbidden. I remembered being about four years old, with my mother, who was dressed in a suit, her thick, dark hair in a long pageboy. There were other people. They were going to do something to me and I was in mortal terror. I was very aware, even at that age, that my mother was emotionally paralyzed, frozen to the spot and was not going to help me. I felt alone, abandoned, alone — so alone. I do not know what happened next. That is as far as my flash of memory took me.

I am shocked that I keep having these small glimpses of things. I always wonder what horror lurks beneath them. I am trying very hard to take care of myself, to turn to God, to write out my anxieties, to soothe myself with music. I go to Al-Anon meetings. I see my therapist. I snuggle up to my husband. I embrace my son. I confide in friends. Little by little I keep on going, I must. Sometimes I feel like the Little Engine That Could, "I think I can. I think I can." One day I may be able to say, "I knew I could."

Janelle M.

THE GIRL INSIDE

I need a place where I can hide
Where I can be
The girl inside.

I need a place where I can stay
A special place
A hideaway.

I need a cove that is lined with moss
And flowers fresh
And pillows soft.

I need a place where I can be
The girl inside
Who is safe and free

I'll rest in guardian angels' arms
And never know
A moment's harm.

Janelle M.

TELLING

Writing about telling is almost as hard as telling.

I had nothing to tell until two years ago. A therapist and a community college in my area cosponsored a weekend workshop on "Women Abused As Children." I knew as I attended that my parents were alcoholics and that I had many symptoms of growing up in that atmosphere. I had figured out about the alcoholism with my own therapist during the previous year of therapy. I thought that was all there was to it.

I was mistaken. Although the experimental work at the workshop gently chipped away at my defenses it was while eating lunch with several women that I was stunned, floored and assaulted with truth. They spoke of having been molested. I said that I was lucky — my grandfather had only kissed and fondled me inappropriately. They were aghast. They said, "You were molested!"

That opened the floodgates. For days I ate, slept and dreamt the ancient events. I was not doing very well. My therapist saw to it that my physician gave me medication to get through this time. In therapy, I talked and talked and talked. I pushed at the fear. It pushed right back.

My therapist advised telling. I had already told my husband and felt horrid and scummy. I was advised to go to my pastor and tell.

I did. It was oh so hard, but I told. He was — of course — loving, caring and nonjudgmental. He advised me to tell our female pastor. And I did. She was supportive of my pain and struggle.

And that, I thought, was that.

But after years of not writing I picked up my pen again. I wrote about my childhood history. I submitted my article and it was accepted for publication. I was so excited I could not sit still. Husband, son, therapist, pastors — all were told of my achievement. But I wanted — needed — more.

So once again I told. I chose a friend I believed I could trust; told her about the article and that the content had to do with my childhood abuse. She accepted me still, did not withdraw, did not judge. Oh, how relieved I was! I will confess to an evening of agony afterwards, questioning my own judgment in telling. But the next time I saw her she asked my husband, "Aren't you excited to have a writer in the family?" I was vindicated.

And by having my previous article in print, I have well and truly told. It is still hard. I still cringe. But these things are part of the fabric of my being, who I am, what I have become. I am alive. I am living, growing and thriving. I have chosen a path calling for courage — and I travel that path each day.

Janelle M.

LISTEN

Listen to me!
I have a voice.
Can you hear me?
No more screaming, shrieking, yelling
No more unreason, terror, fright
Do not give me your boundless needs
Your vast demands
Your aching void.
For I was just a little child
I am that child still
Hiding in a woman's body.
Other people reach out
Teach me about safety
And dignity
And respect.

Listen to me!
I have a voice.

Janelle M.

LIVING OUT LOUD

I wrote to them today.
I put it in a story.
But the subject was me
And I put it on paper
And now they know.
They know.

I pray for myself.
In words and in song.
I said it.
I did it.
They know.

They may have known long ago.
They didn't protect me.
That was their job.
They failed.
They know.

And now I must learn to live
Out loud with words
That can't be taken back.

I was molested by my grandfather.
And now my parents know.
They know.

Janelle M.

BUILDING

Brick by brick
Stone by stone
I build the wall
That will be my home.
Build it high
Build it strong
Build it thick
And build it long.

Janelle M.

A PROGRESS REPORT ON JANELLE

Right now I am recovering memories — again — and my healing seems to be progressing with the help of therapy and Al-Anon. Sometimes I wonder when I will ever come to the end of this; but through this difficult time I have a sense of God being by my side supporting and upholding me.

I have been in group therapy for eight months now. I just began individual therapy with a new therapist three months ago. My life has its ups and downs but it holds promise. Music, writing and my spiritual life continue to offer much solace.

I have been in therapy for over four years with a solid, stable (I really like solid and stable) male therapist. I am still working on my "issues" and feel privileged to be able to do so. I did not ever expect to feel as healthy and happy as this. There is still plenty of recovery and I see it as a lifetime process, but hey, what else am I doing with the rest of my life? I have been attending Al-Anon meetings and fit right in with the other people who are adult children of alcoholics. Since I never anticipated fitting in anywhere, it is an absolute pleasure. Also, the creative juices are once again flowing and I am feeling free to write.

My Dream

A feeling comes back to me, something from a long time ago. It was when I was a child. I had a dream, a special dream that I clung to, that I clung to desperately. I remember I would go off by myself for hours and dream my little childhood dream. You see, as long as my dream lived inside of me I could live, I could survive it all with my little dream.

In my dream my father was not beating my mother until she was all bloody. He was not saying, "You bitch, you whore, I'm going to kill you!" Words that sent shivers up my spine. And no, I did not hear her screams . . . everyday. Screams that still echo in my mind, that still leave me paralyzed with fear, that still haunt me. No, that was not in my dream.

In my dreams my father was not taking me by the hand and leading me up those stairs (Oh, God, not again) that led to his bedroom, while my mother and sisters went out shopping. No, he did not take my clothes off and sit me on the edge of the bed as he knelt down before me. My eyes were not squeezed tightly, my teeth were not gritted hard, I did not numb out. No, I am sure that was not in my dream.

In my dream my father was not dragging my sister across the floor by her hair in front of his friends. No, he did not make her kiss the floor in front of them. They did not just sit there watching, saying nothing, as through the years so many would do . . . including our mother. Just watching, watching the violence, watching our fear, pain, humiliations and the tears in our eyes, never saying anything, never offering their hand, just watching. And no, in my dream I was not awakened, like every other night, to the thundering of my father's voice and to the sounds of glass breaking. I was not lying in my bed, trembling, my teeth chattering, literally paralyzed with fear and unable to move, as my sisters rushed off to "save" our mother's life once again. No, that was not in my dream.

In my dream my father did not come get me out of bed late at night. That could not have happened . . . and where was my mom? He did not take me up to his bed and take my panties off and put them under my mother's pillow, just as he had done so many times before. I did not slowly reach my hand up under the pillow and grasp my panties tightly in my little hand. I did not clutch them for dear life. Somehow having them in my possession, hanging on to them, somehow made me feel safer. And no, he did not pull my nightgown up and put his . . . no, that was not in my dream.

In my dream my father was not pushing that horribly scary thing (to a child's mind and to a child's body) in and out of me. His huge strong hand holding both of my tiny ones in his grasp. His words, spoken with icy danger, "Shh! . . . Do not move . . . be still . . . shh," still haunt me. I did not move again. I simply floated away. I went far away, and no, I did not move again. I am sure that was not in my dream either.

In my dream this insecure, irrational man was not here by my side, controlling my life, destroying everything precious to me, inside of me. I was not, for some reason I can not quite understand, unable to say no to him, unable to get him out of my life, and unable to hate him without loving him and wanting desperately to please him.

This man, this man who "loves me," does not have me pinned down and is not hitting me over and over in the face. He is not throwing me against walls and he is not choking me, and no, he is not saying, "You bitch, you whore, I am going to kill you!" No, those words are not ringing loudly in my head, striking something very familiar in me, something from a long time ago. No, this man next to me, who represents everything that I despise, was not in my dream.

In my dream I was not getting my knife out and sharpening it, as I had done many times before. I did not then savagely cut my arm up, driven by some mysterious force, all the while saying, "You bitch, you whore, I hate you!" over and over. No, I did not look down at my bloody arm, as if it was not a part of me, and wonder why I felt nothing but satisfaction. No, I am sure that was not in my dream either.

Somewhere along the way, maybe from too much pain, from too many scars that never seem to heal, or from too much sadness and emptiness, that dream that lived inside of me quietly died, unnoticed. I lost that dream to a peaceful place, a calm and quiet place. I know that I will once again know my dream. I will finally live my dream as it lived inside of me through all those years of hell.

Dina C.

SILENCE

Darkness creeping
    Children screaming
Mouths crying out
    With no voices
Silent screams
    Amidst the darkness
Silent terror
    In the night
The screams are not heard
    For they have no sound
Though we know that they are there
    We ignore the screams
        And only hear the
        Silence . . .

Dina C.

A PROGRESS REPORT ON DINA

The one way I have found to get my feelings and emotions out is to write. If my poems make people feel something, then I know I have written something good. I hope that they can help someone else.

I have recently gotten out of an emotionally and physically abusive relationship. I am trying very hard to learn to like myself again and to regain some level of self-esteem and self-worth. I am an agoraphobic, just one of the ways my childhood experiences have affected me. I have found the mental health system to be totally ignorant of the dynamics of child sexual, physical and emotional abuse. I am actively involved with our local Humane Society and in the past year and a half have taken in over 150 abused, neglected and abandoned animals. Not only do I have strong feelings and views on childhood sexual abuse, but also on the issues of domestic violence. That women are being stabbed, shot or beaten to death by their mates is unacceptable.

WHO ARE YOU?

Who are you?
We know you by the deeds you do;
You labor and toil
While many lives you soil.
Admired for your generosity
Your actions are an atrocity.
Respected church and civic leader
Your crimes a felony, not a misdemeanor.

Who are you?
If others only knew.
Doing what you want, not should,
Calling it love, calling it good.
Oh, the secrets that you keep,
Souls deprived of innocence you keep.
The morality and piety you profess
Hide carnal lusts you won't confess.

Smile your smile of guile
You escaped justice for a while,
To be judged by God above
For your deeds of perverse love.
Forgiveness is a must,
But you I can never trust
Gemini, you deceive
Which of your faces can I believe?
Who are you?

D. Leslie

EVIL

Evil comes in many forms
Evil wears many faces
When evil appears good
Evil is most dangerous.

D. Leslie

A PROGRESS REPORT ON D. LESLIE

Although my molester was never convicted, he did enter therapy. Because he was able to keep everything secret, his reputation in the community and at church and at work remain intact, except for the few who know. The fact that he basically got away with it caused me the most pain. I spent a few years feeling either angry or numb. Now I can express my feelings and get on with my life regardless of what happens to him, thanks to support from my husband and sister who endured more abuse.

EXPECTATION

Standing quietly, lost in thought
daydreaming out the window and savoring
this miracle of late fertility,
this gift of resurrection.
Unconsciously, I've clasped my hands
lightly beneath my middle
in a classic pregnant stance.
Remembering, perhaps,
the children I've already borne,
the sweet delicious secret of their being
before their birth.
When they were mine, and mine alone.
A tiny seed of hope embedded deeply
soon to grow.
I feel the life that stirs within me
Reminiscence and anticipation blend
Sensations, both new and familiar,
Ripe with possibility, lush with potential,
wonder and delight at nurturing another soul
within myself.
Pregnancy agrees with me,
a nearly perfect state of being.
And now again, I shelter seed
To grow a child, to grow a woman . . .
Pregnant with myself.
A microscopic cell of hope
for rebirth of the child I lost
Stillborn or aborted by despair
So long ago,
Miraculously revived to live again.
This time I will protect her, keep her safe
And raise her proud and strong.
I feel the flutter of her hand,
the warmth of life.
As real to me as a physical being,
This fetus of the heart.

Doris D.

A PROGRESS REPORT ON DORIS

I am thirty-nine years old. I am a police dispatcher and mother of four sons, ages fifteen, seventeen, nineteen and twenty-one. I was sexually abused at eight or nine years of age by a neighbor. Although I have suffered from anxiety attacks, sleep disorders and various nervous conditions throughout my life, I was not aware of the abuse until two years ago when a set of similar circumstances triggered the memory. I have been alternately hysterical, nonfunctional and irrational since. With the help of a wonderful therapist, the support of my husband and children, and a regimen of anti-anxiety medication, I am coming to terms with my memories. It is through poetry and short essays that I have been able to express some of what I feel and dispel some of the rage. Although remembering, talking and writing about it is very painful for me, it has also helped me to understand my behavior and my lack of self-esteem. I've got a long way to go yet, but I have more good days all the time.

REMEMBERING

There are times, usually most of the time, that I pretend that everything is okay. The dimly remembered fears are dream-like and distant, not real or to be dealt with. Then there are those moments when my body remembers, even though my mind doesn't. I am forced to deal with the overwhelming reality of my abuse manifested as pure terror in the pit of my stomach. Tears pouring down my face and the voice of my little girl inside saying over and over, "I wanna go home. I am afraid. I am so afraid. Please let me go home now." Then I breathe, and remember that I am grown up now. There is only this moment, here and now, and that I can't be hurt all over again. I breathe, and breathe in hope and breathe out fear. I remember that I am big now, and can take care of my little girl.

I offer up the shame of remembering on the altar of my survivorship. I remind myself that I am healing, one step at a time, at my own pace and in my own way. Even as I set these words down I break silence. I claim my life as my own. I claim all of it — the fear, the pain and the shame, so I can claim all the joy and the letting go as well.

One step at a time. One moment to each second. One breath for each fear — one prayer for each hour: These are the thoughts that carry me through the anxiety and the terror of remembering.

Catherine C.

SEEING THE DARKNESS
BEFORE THE LIGHT:
Insights And Perceptions

And so the journey intensifies. Certain sounds, smells, places, or media presentations may trigger some unwanted memories or inexplicable fears. Memory may come gradually and sometimes only in fleeting glimpses. You may not be able to identify the memories until they hit you full force. Either way, it is important to accept what comes.

At one time numbness was all you felt; now you are feeling all the emotions intertwined with memories of abuse. This is the hardest part of recovery. It demands that you look inside the very core of your being and face your greatest fear — the reality of your abuse. Until now, your abuse might have been denied, minimized, stored away, or camouflaged; that is no longer possible.

Sometimes the memory seems as real as the experience itself. Although the feelings are intense, realize that you can control them. Remember, that was then and this is now. During your abuse, you were experiencing the effects of an intolerable situation. As a child you could not express the feelings that accompanied your personal terror. Now the hurt, anger, confusion, hate, humiliation, and a multitude of other feelings reverberate through your life. When you experience these emotions, you may feel as if you are once again in a victimization cycle. Know that this will pass.

As feelings emerge, it is healing to allow their expression. They may feel like an underground volcano waiting to erupt, but you should not try to repress them. You must create a safe way to vent your feelings, however overwhelming and frightening they may seem. You will feel lighter after releasing some of the intensity; however, not do attempt this process by yourself. I encourage you to get involved in recovery groups, joining with others who are experiencing similar struggles.

Reliving memories of your abuse and attaching new emotions to them is draining, so take extra care of yourself physically as well as emotionally. Take naps, soak in the tub, listen to peaceful music, journal, find some healthy physical activity to help diffuse this powerful energy. Allow yourself to be whoever you need to be. Nurture yourself and remember: You are not alone in this process.

Wendy Ann Wood

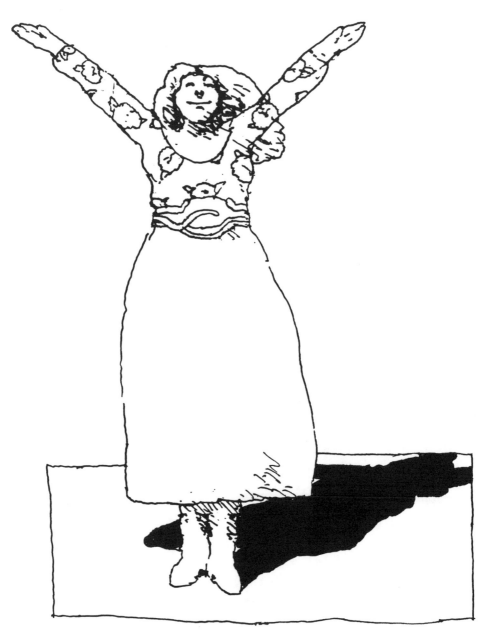

CHAPTER THREE

MOVING BEYOND
THE DARKNESS

TELLING ABOUT IT

You stumble on words a lot and your thoughts ramble.
You stutter and your stomach feels like
    you want to throw up.
You forget to end sentences — forget to breathe —
    and you talk real fast, trying to make your words
    keep up with your mind — until you say a word
    that sticks in your throat —
    and fear takes over
and your mind goes numb and you mumble some more
    wishing you never even began talking
        about IT.
All of your fears still connected
    and you wonder who you can trust.
But still,
    words keep coming out of your mouth.
There's this unexplainable feeling
    that if you don't tell right NOW
    you'll never again tell anyone
        about IT.

Your body hurts where you hurt as a child
and you wonder why the bruises and cuts
don't show on the outside when you can
feel them all so painfully inside.

You start remembering and telling about things
    you thought you had forgotten
The nightmares start up again
    and sleeping with a light on becomes comforting.
You feel sad — frustrated — confused — guilty —
    disgusted — victimized — depressed
        and angry.

You yell a lot and you cry. You throw things
and you hit a lot of pillows, screaming out your hurt —

   or,

you curl into a small ball;
your throat tightens, and your fear
is so overwhelming, that all you can do is whisper.
There's an incredible feeling of wanting to run —
of wanting to be busy with other things —
yet knowing that only by talking
      about IT
will your fears and hurt go away.

So, you keep telling
You realize you can't deny
what happened any longer. It's a part of who you are,
of why you respond the way you do
    to love and touch.

IT becomes a part of what makes you unique
and also part of your strength;
as the realization comes that
you are not a frightened child — hurt and unsure —
but an adult — capable and strong.
You know how and when you want to say, "NO,"
and when you want to say, "YES."
Then you take some deep breaths and try to relax,
   because you know that telling
      about IT
   will be easier the next time.

Jill

A PROGRESS REPORT ON JILL

For years, I have been learning to get in touch with my anger over being sexually abused. I beat pillows — I screamed and cried. But not until I could get beyond the anger and forgive those who abused me, did I experience any inner feeling. Though it didn't come easily, I was able to not only have forgiveness for them, but to truly love them.

At this time in my life, through my church, I am working with teenage girls who have drug- or alcohol-related problems. I am co-facilitating an ongoing support group for women who were sexually abused as children. We offer them hope and healing through prayer and encouragement.

I am working towards establishing an ongoing support and information group for teenage girls who have been sexually and physically abused.

MEMORIES AND SECRETS
Letters Between Mother And Daughter

My dear daughter,

All your life I treated you and your sister as individuals, always trying to impress upon you to develop your separate talents, to never cease enlarging your minds. Both of you have extremely twisted and incorrect memories of your childhood. No mother ever was prouder of her children. All those years when I worked like four people, I never ceased to have pride in myself and my two wonderful children. I was so proud of my two little girls. It did not matter to me what the sex. They were my own. If you remember, I have said, "I will fight to the death for my own."

Your father started working after school at fourteen — he gave what he earned to his widowed mother. He came to Washington at eighteen, as a messenger boy, went to school nights to earn a degree in accounting — still sending money to his mother. After he died at thirty-eight, when I was disposing of his things, I was appalled at the waste of his young life — he had worked so hard and wanted so desperately to get ahead. Yes, he had pride in himself.

Be proud that you are descended from some of the most handsome and most progressive nationalities on earth — pure Celt (Scottish); the great, talented, realistic French (and as you know, Oh Lord, how proud they are of themselves — also smart — they want to keep France French); and English-Welsh. Be proud of that heritage. Is this being racist? I am a reader of history.

I know what is happening to America and the white race all over the world, but particularly here. Before your life is over you will see what I mean. The white race is committing suicide. White women are refusing to have their own children. The people with the best minds are refusing to have their own children. You'd better think about these things I have said, now and previous to this time.

As one grows older all one has to look forward to is a future in one's grandchildren. Yes, I produced, and you could produce "prime specimens." If your father had been older than I and had been able to acquire some financial security before marriage, I would definitely have had at least one other child, regardless of its sex. I wanted my children so much.

You cannot imagine what it is like to have children for a man who does not want them. Although I never regretted your birth, I wanted a boy. The generations cannot be cast aside. I have been punished terribly because I did not honor and go to my mother — even though she was terribly cruel and jealous of me when I was growing up. I remember when my girls were only eighteen, before my world crashed about my head — my darling girls. No woman ever loved her children more than I, but there is a limit to what one will accept even from one's own children. This is the last letter I shall write you, unless I hear from you. I have been bruised over the last ten years. I cannot take much more

I received the pretty shell box. I hope you made it. Part of my grief about you, except I wish you were close, is that I believe you are neglecting all of your artistic talents. About "liking" what you are, I always thought you a wonderful, brilliant child; but as a mother I cannot help worrying about your future.

If you ever get pregnant, please do not destroy your child. I would even help you raise it. If you destroy it, when you are old you will bitterly regret it. A child should be greeted with joy. I always stood by you and wanted you to have advantages that I had not had, although my parents did the same for me. I really loved being with you and wanted more time with you than I had. I am sorry you had to be latchkey kids.

You'd better think about the things I have said, now and previous to this time. I am nearly seventy-two years old, a diabetic who must take care of myself to prevent complications, and my eyesight is failing. I am developing a cataract on one eye. I wonder, after all these years, forgetting the above sentence, what one woman is supposed to put up with. I faced the things that happened to me, accepting my life and whatever responsibilities that entailed, and went on. One has to accept life, no life is perfect. My God, I was an innocent. I really thought I gave you a happy childhood, and, above all, I trusted you and your sister implicitly. I have found out, here and there, that trust was mislaid.

Yes, I am nearly seventy-two years old, and even if late, have been trying to make a life for myself which is more ME. At last I have had time to make a few friends, which I never had time for while you were growing up. I know now I was wrong to give of myself to that extent — but I never thought it would cause you and your sister to dislike me so much. I never intended to hang on to you in any way. If you remember correctly (the evidence indicates that you do not) I tried to help each of you develop your distinctive talents, realizing that you were such different individuals. I am appalled at how you have destroyed yourself — don't blame it on your childhood. Your father died, yes, and it was a devastating experience when you were seven. Do you not know it was for me too, especially that I had to leave my children and go to work? But, how I tried, and gave myself to make up for that fact. Whether you and your sister have any respect for those years, I respect myself for them. I wonder how many present-day women will respect themselves when they are seventy-two years old. But, then, women today no longer believe in that kind of commitment.

You have always been practically a genius, my dear. I have always known you could be a fine artist or almost anything you put your mind to. Whatever problems you have developed after you left home — obviously to put as many miles between you and me as possible — you did to yourself. For fifteen years I have been fighting depression because of my daughter's lack of love for me, and worrying over you and what you were doing to yourself. If what I am is what has disturbed you, then that is just too bad. I was never anything but good to you. It would seem that you might at least let me have a little peace in my last good years.

Your main problem, possibly, is you realize you have wasted your beautiful youth. Well, nothing can be done about that, but you can accept the fact and stop blaming your childhood for it. The years are inexorable. How well I know. And your father, who had the whole burden of his mother and younger brothers put on his shoulders at fourteen years of age, never stopped loving her and his family.

I have made many mistakes concerning my life, I know, but one goes on, and I do not blame others for my mistakes in judgment. But my main drive in life was to see that you missed nothing because of your father's death and to give you advantages I did not have. You are extremely beautiful, extremely intelligent and

talented. I was happy when I learned you were studying art because I always knew you were artistic, and that you had stopped
smoking and were jogging — I hope you have not stopped these
activities.

I remember so many sweet things about you and shall always
love the lovely girl you have been. You did not have a bad childhood. I did my very best for you. When, if ever, you are able to communicate with me as a daughter should, I am ready and willing to
hear from you. You'd better think about the things I have said, now
and previous to this time.

As ever, with love,
Mother

Mother,

Your words twisted my childhood memories into terrible secrets, secrets even unto myself. Your words always told me you
knew me better than I knew myself — and I believed you. Your
words turned my child-molester father into an angel called early to
heaven. Your words glorified our ancient past for the wrong reasons. Your words taught me to hate others in order to feel superior.
Your words taught me to hate myself.

Your words endlessly threatened me. Your words created a world
of isolation which separated us from the rest of the world. Your
words told me life was imperfect without a man — no matter how
imperfect the man. Your words belied the reality that you did not
want me, and your act of attempted infanticide. Your words inti-
mated I was the cause of your suffering and I would be punished.

Your words tried to erase my memories of traumatic events.
Your words never gave without taking away. Your words convinced
me to abort to keep another from experiencing what I had. I did
not then know I could break the chain. Your words substituted love
for other things.

Your words clouded your vision — created a world you could
accept. Your words turned the slightest mischief into a capital
crime. Your words accused me of your own transgressions against

yourself. Your words enforced a remembering that was correct only to you. Your words of incessant encouragement buried my creativity along with my true feelings. One cannot exist without the other.

Your words attempted to eradicate your guilt and complicity. Your words would not accept whatever respect and gratitude I did have for you. Your words were ludicrous when speaking of trust and commitment. Your words made me afraid of trying any endeavor, for fear I would not live up to your expectations. Your words projected on me your own inadequacies.

Your words were sometimes wise out of context. Your words contradicted themselves. Your words claimed ownership of my victories. Your words convoluted, perverted, entangled, maimed, and buried me. Your words were never a two-way communication device.

Renee

I Was Twenty-Five And A Child

Some women are fortunate enough to know at an early age that their family is different. But not I. Not until years of trying to fit into a strange mold, years of nonaffection, years of unhappiness — trying to figure out what it was about ME that was so wrong. After a year of professional analysis I found out the truth — that it was they who were strange and not I.

All of my life I have been an intelligent, capable, strong and lovable woman who experienced time and again empty and abusive relationships with men. I felt no inner courage when faced with job challenges. I solved problems by running. I was frightened when I left the security of my room, felt claustrophobic in crowds, agoraphobic on a deserted beach. I never strayed too far from the nearest bathroom. I felt like a maniac in the presence of a man. I was never satisfied or happy just to be alive.

In a rare moment of intimacy my mother shared the circumstances of my birth. Picture a maternity home in the late '40s, a midwife and a country doctor are present. My father is in the room. My mother is eighteen years old and totally ignorant of the birthing process. It must have been the transition phase of labor when the pains are most intense and the emotional toll was the greatest, as she began to scream in terror that she was going to die. My father ran out of the room. The doctor administered ether and soon I was born.

Born into a world of screams and anger for causing such pain. There was no warm welcoming committee for me. My earliest memories are of loneliness, searching for affection and warmth and looking for smiles of approval. I received instead messages of, "It would certainly be easier for us if you did not exist. Do this or do that for us. Stay out of the way. Be quiet. Do not make any demands." In essence, "Do not exist."

No wonder I found it difficult, if not impossible, to build a positive self-image. No wonder that I jumped with instant adulation toward anyone who would show me the least amount of attention or affection without knowing whether it was healthy or not. I only knew that it was attention and that it felt good, almost narcotic.

How ready I was for a Catholic priest to bestow his graces of attention, recognition, and physical affection. I was twelve and a half years of age and so desperately lonely and starving for affection. During a rehearsal for a May Crowning of the Virgin Mary, he caught my eye and mouthed the words, "I love you." I blinked my eyes, so sure was I that I was seeing a vision. He repeated the words, "I love you." Then he dismissed the group. I was the last to leave. He grabbed me and hugged me and tried to kiss me. God, I thought, this man loves me. I was overwhelmed with a rush of feelings that I cannot even now label. I rushed out of the room, my heart racing. Since no parents were at the rehearsal he drove us all home, leaving me the last one to deliver. After insisting I sit next to him in the car, he pulled me over to the middle of the front seat. Before I could protest, his hand was between my legs and fumbling for my vagina.

Thus began thirteen years of weekly molestation by a respected and powerful man who was a Catholic priest in a quiet Midwestern farming community. I was betrayed by an adult man that I trusted.

The incredibly devious and subtle way in which he manipulated his way into our family was indeed criminal. Into the midst of rural poverty and social ignorance he brought gifts of clothing, food, and trips to movies, concerts and plays. He skillfully orchestrated situations in which he could, unobserved, fondle and touch, manipulate and caress the sexual organs of all the girls in my household.

After many months of agonizing fear and almost paralyzing aloneness, I left home and the clutches of this priest who was rapidly suffocating me.

I was twenty-five and a child. I bounced from relationship to relationship, leaving each one emotionally drained to nothingness. Into my emotional desert came a flood of anger that decimated what was left of my spirit. The self-destructive nature of anger alerted me to seek professional help. I learned that many victims of childhood sexual molestation follow a pattern throughout their lives. My life seemed to be a carbon copy of that pattern. My rage manifested itself in flight behavior, unsuccessful relationships with men, excessive use of drugs and alcohol, compulsive eating, inexplicable outbursts of anxiety and anger, abysmally low self-esteem and very little self-confidence.

Through the fine expertise of one woman counselor, I began to raise some serious questions. Why was I so susceptible at twelve and a half years of age? Why did I feel so powerless to fight off the molestations of a priest? Why did I feel so responsible for the disease that infected me and my whole family?

Through the painful dredging of buried memories I discovered I had been sexually molested by two male cousins when I was six years of age, that I had been sexually molested in elementary school by older boys, that I had been sexually molested by my own grandfather as early as five years of age. A shocking and lonely truth blasted my present reality. My own mother had been aware of my sexual molestation by my cousins. Both her behavior toward me and also her attitude, then and now, implied that she blamed me. Why did my mother not protect me? Was she also a victim of childhood sexual molestation? Had she internalized the feelings that women were to be used by men for whatever purpose whenever they chose? Was she too frightened to speak out? Would anyone have listened? After the birth of my sister in the late '50s, my mother suffered an overwhelming depression. She sought help in a sanitarium in which her only treatment was electric shock.

Unbeknownst to me, I had been suffering both her pain and also my own for all those years. Had she been able to solve her own victimization as a child, she would not have carried it over to me by being overprotective, acting like a doormat, and being silent when she saw someone abusing her own daughter. It was no wonder that I was almost catatonic with rage.

Curiosity led me to inquire into the whereabouts of the priest who sexually molested me and my sisters. Imagine the feelings I had when I discovered that he was not dead, that he had not resigned or retired. Rather, he was alive and well and functioning as a Catholic priest in another Midwestern farming community.

I reported him to his Archbishop. The following is the letter that I sent:

Dear Archbishop,

My name is _____. I am currently involved in a therapy/support group for women who have been molested as children. I was molested by a Catholic priest when I was thirteen years of age. This priest is currently functioning in your archdiocese. His name is _____ and he is the pastor of _____ Parish. I am very concerned because I fear that he may be molesting children and/or women today.

To document further: From July 1960 until fall 1972, _____ sexually molested me at these locations: rest areas along various highways and in movie theaters across the state.

During my high school years of 1960 – 1964, _____ molested me weekly in the kitchen of my parents' home (under the pretense of helping me with my homework), on the way to music lessons, in the Catholic church choir loft and attic, and the Catholic grade school.

Isolated incidents occurred in my own bedroom and in my parents' home (while it was being painted with paint _____ had purchased for the project), in the rectory, in the basement of the grade school, and in a motel room in Canada.

I am reporting this to you — not to press charges against this priest but to inform you that he has in the past molested me and my sisters and may be molesting someone today. I would like to save one person from the emotional and spiritual pain that I have suffered for the last twenty years.

My family was incredibly poor and socially isolated. There were ten children on a struggling farm. He took advantage of our extreme poverty and of the naiveté and social ignorance of my parents. We were flattered, proud, and felt blessed that a Catholic priest of God was visiting our home and showering us with gifts, praise and attention.

Our parish needed a choir director and an organist. _____ offered to pay for my music lessons which afforded him the opportunity to have me alone with him weekly. To further ease the financial burden of my parents, he bought clothes, shoes, birthday presents for my brothers and sisters. He paid for most of my college education and bought me clothes and cars.

Throughout this time period, there were countless opportunities for him to be alone with me or my younger sisters, and he was often dressed as a priest representing God and His Holy Church. He would say such things as, "It's okay, I'm not going to hurt you. I'm a priest. I'll teach you about these things. I love you."

After struggling for years to break away from the powerful dependency trap I was in, I left home in 1973 at which time _____ increased his molestation of my sisters.

My parents, by this time fearful, inadequate, confused, and aware of the betrayal of a priest they had once respected and trusted, tried to break off all contact with _____. In a fit of alcoholic anger, he publicly embarrassed them from the pulpit. He shamed and insulted them in front of the whole congregation, forcing my mother to leave the service in tears. Still faithful, however, my parents joined another Catholic church in the area.

I have prayed and sought much counsel in the preparation of this letter. Had I found out that _____ was not alive, or was retired and receiving extensive help for his problems, I would not have sought your help in this matter. The fact that he is functioning today as a priest and as a representative of the Catholic church bothers me a great deal.

Please investigate this matter and respond.

Editor's Note: Several letters have been exchanged between this author and the Archbishop. His last letter to her stated: "I can tell you that I spoke with _____. He assures me that nothing of this nature has happened since the times indicated in your letter. Also, there is no evidence whatsoever to indicate that there has been a problem these past years. I believe _____ is telling the truth. As you may surmise, _____ is approaching the age of retirement. He will be seventy years old shortly. I hope the above information puts your mind at rest."

After receiving this letter the author wrote a letter to her offender which reads as follows (with a few deletions of repetitive material):

D_{ear} _____,

As I collect my thoughts to write this letter to you, I am bombarded with so many different thoughts and feelings that I find it almost impossible to put into words what I am now feeling and thinking about what happened to me beginning the summer of my thirteenth year.

By now you know that I have reported you to your Archbishop. You sexually molested me for thirteen years until I left home in 1972. I am only writing to you now because this is one more step that I must and want to take in my own healing process.

The emotional and physical trauma that I felt as a child can be compared to the physical and emotional trauma felt by some Vietnam War vets who are now experiencing the affects of war and Agent Orange on their spirits and on their bodies. Like the various forms of cancer showing up in their bodies, so too, the trauma of your abuse has taken its toll on me and my whole life, up to and including this time, even today as I write this letter.

I trusted you, a priest, a man of God. I idolized you and your dynamic charisma that seemed to be doing so much good for people, the Church and for God! You were thirty years older than I! How could you use your hand, anointed with Holy Oil, to fondle and caress my breasts, to manipulate and to masturbate my vagina? How can you justify that behavior with your vocation as a priest of the Holy Roman Catholic Church?

I was not the only child you molested. My sisters have come forth to acknowledge your attempts and successes. There were others outside my family.

How could you ever imagine that you were doing me or any child a favor by sexually molesting us? Sexual molestation is legally defined as any sexual contact with a child or the use of a child for the sexual gratification of someone else. It includes the fondling of the genitals, or asking the child to do so, oral sex and attempts to penetrate the vagina or anus.

You, and your sick tendency to seek intimate nonjudgmental, affectionate relationships with children have nearly ruined my whole life! I trusted you and you violated that trust! Never since that time have I been able to form a lasting, healthy, trusting relationship with a man. During the most formative years of my life, when I should have been forming healthy, normal attitudes about my own sexuality, you chose to "teach me about sex" by forcing me to masturbate you, by manipulating me into situations where you could sexually molest me, by using bribery and friendship to get me to sexually satisfy you, and by using threats to enforce secrecy. I was so afraid then, and so concerned to protect my parents, my brothers and sisters, and to protect you, that I allowed this abuse to continue for so long.

You sensed a weakness in our family structure, you knew my parents were poor, and socially backward, timid, and in awe of you. YOU TOOK ADVANTAGE OF THIS! YOU MOLESTED ME AND MY SISTERS! AND YOU LIED ABOUT IT!

For your own purposes you planted in me the seeds of open rebellion, hatred, and distrust of my own parents — the only people who could have helped me, had they known the truth.

So many physical and emotional side-effects are still with me — my fear of closed-in areas, my fear of large luxury model cars, my fear of men, my anxiety attacks, my agoraphobia . . . I have not been able to sing for over ten years or sit and play the piano. I have the paralyzing fear that someone will come up from behind me and molest me as I sit down to practice.

You did me no favors by buying me clothes, music lessons, college or cars. You took away my childhood and my adolescence. You molested me when I was powerless to defend myself.

Within two weeks of receiving this letter, I want you to write a formal letter of apology signed by yourself and witnessed by your Archbishop. I want you to address this letter to my family and in it to apologize for the damage you inflicted on me and them. I want you to seek professional help for yourself.

In conclusion, I want to call your attention to Matthew 18: 6 and 10. "But who so shall offend one of these little ones which believe in Me, it were better for him that a millstone were hanged about his neck, and that he were drowned to the depths of the sea."

I am now thirty-nine and an adolescent. I am piecing together a new life based on the knowledge that I am truly lovable, capable and strong. Knowing the truth has helped to set me free from my paralyzing past. I am learning how to trust, how to think, how to feel and how to assert my rights.

Anonymous

A PROGRESS REPORT ON THIS AUTHOR

I searched for and found a feminist attorney who helped me to compose a demand letter and to sue the Catholic priest for damages. After six to nine months of long distance correspondence she and I succeeded in demanding and obtaining a sum of money from him! This sum in no way compensates for the years of delayed stress from his sexual assault but it gave me a feeling of closure to nearly three years of individual and group therapy.

Breaking the silence about his molestation of me, and my reporting him to the Child Abuse Registry as well as to his archbishop, and my demanding some restitution through a legal channel, has helped me to reclaim my sense of power.

Three more steps that I want to add to my present recovery process include:

1. To mend my spirituality, by finding a spiritual community.
2. To lose the weight of fat and "anger" my body carries.
3. To join a mixed support group.

To Love Myself

WHY was it so hard?
So hard to wrap my arms around myself
To love myself for all that I am,
For all that I might be.

WHY was it so hard?
To accept the hurt and crying child,
To let her know it was all right
To feel and to be.

WHY was it so hard?
So hard to feel that she was a welcome and wondrous
Part, to treasure her wide-eyed innocence,
And unwavering trust of the heart.

WHY was it so hard?
So hard to realize that she alone could view the world,
As fresh and new each day,
To appreciate her gloriously
Curious way

WHY was it so hard?
So hard to truly love myself,
For all that I am,
For all that I might be.
So hard to believe,
That she, after all,

Is ME.

Karen S.

SURVIVORS' GROUP

What does it mean to be an adult survivor of child abuse? It means looking in the mirror and seeing garbage, if you see anything at all. It means finding ways to numb yourself so you don't have to feel or think. It means being afraid to go asleep in the dark, or without a weapon at hand. It means waking night after night because of nightmares or because you sense evil in your room. It means thinking that you are crazy because sane people sleep in the dark and are not afraid of things that go bump in the night. It means keeping yourself so busy that your head is full of static-white noise that drowns out the screaming child that lives inside you.

We sat that first Monday evening in a large, softly lighted room, some dozen women who had come together uneasily if not reluctantly, to speak of our dirty little secrets. In the following weeks our tales were told in bits and pieces. They were terrifying stories of abuse by fathers, grandfathers, mothers, uncles, cousins, brothers, friends, neighbors. We cried and shook. Our backs and bellies hurt. We felt we might suffocate. We clenched our teeth. We were cold, hot, raw, vulnerable, angry, sad, and afraid. We comforted and confronted each other with hugs, laughter, honesty and the recognition of shared experiences. We felt safe.

We found that we had dealt with our particular pain in ways that numbed us and still allowed us to go on more or less well. Some of us forgot, repressed what had happened to us and are only now remembering. That makes us feel crazy, but we are not. Some of us have misused drugs and alcohol. That makes us feel weak but we are not. We have continued to abuse our own bodies and spirits years after the other horror has stopped. That makes us feel bad, but we are not.

So we came together to think about ourselves; to try to find the person inside each of us who is truly our own, that self, free of our defensiveness, that enables us to survive. We came together and said to each other, "You are not alone. You are not crazy, you are not vile, dirty or defective. You had no control over what happened to you, it was not your fault." And we said, "You are good. You are clean and bright. You are lovable. You are loved." We learned to believe it.

Suzanne C.

BROKEN PIECES

I sleep with my kitty — little Mau. She is my child, my friend, my littlest love. She meets me at the gate whenever I come home and rolls on her back so I can rub her tummy. I think that Mau loves me too — and that's so special. When I take a nap on the sofa, she curls up on my chest to sleep. She gets pissed off if I move, glares for a moment, closes her eyes and falls back to sleep. Sometimes I wake up at night in a panic — Mau is sleeping between my legs and I feel crowded, tense, invaded. I move her quickly and close up my legs. I feel bad — she thinks it's comfortable there and I make her move. She loves me, I think; but that doesn't mean I have to let her be close to me everywhere. With Mau, I can say no.

I have been sick this week, stayed home from work. It's been a relief, not facing the hatred, the silence, the wall of isolation. I do good work (I know I do — I don't give myself compliments easily). I took this job in a wild grasp for stability. Steady paycheck. Consistent work. A job I could leave at the end of the day, to have time to think, to identify feelings. But then the wall was built and I felt trapped. I am scared of this feeling that I've had before; and I wonder if all the feelings come back to the old one. Maybe nothing changes, it just gets bigger. I feel sad. So I'm home from work, hiding in my home with Mau, feeling safe, feeling trapped, reaching out every few hours to assure myself that I'm not alone.

I went to the doctor this week because it was so hard to breathe. I asked a friend to take me, because I was in pain, because I was scared. The doctor had to put his hands on me before passing judgment. "You are sick, I can hear how hard it is for you to breathe." Relief. He believed me — I'm really sick. I am not faking, I am not crazy, it was okay to see a doctor this time. It's okay to feel pain, this time — it's real.

It was very different, the last time I saw my therapist. I spoke of things I never mentioned before. I made connections I was always afraid of. I talked about suicide in a new way, wanting to be listened to, so the deciding times didn't hurt so much. I talked about different pain — my uncle, my brother, the doctors, my mother, my friends. I talked of feeling crazy and different, and all alone. I told her of the time I learned that people liked themselves, and what a shock it was. I hurt so bad — it was something everyone knew but me.

I wanted to cry as all these memories tumbled out. But I don't really cry. I wanted her to hold me, but I didn't want to ask, I was afraid she might. I might cry if she did. I made up jokes to ease the pain and the flow of pictures rushing into my head. All my memories were connected to different houses and states, that was how I remembered. I wanted that to be funny, so it would hurt less. She told me what I went through was bad, and it was understandable that I was so tired. I think it's the first time I ever heard that. The pain was real; I am not crazy, not faking it — it's real pain. I left feeling very different, like something important happened. I wanted to call her and tell her but I didn't.

Mommy, I don't want to feel bad for what they did to me. I don't want to remember hands on little girl's secret places that I didn't understand. I don't want to remember being too little to be touched too hard. I don't want to remember those games and big fights. I don't want to remember threats for fighting back. I don't want to remember being dragged out of the closet to visit relatives I was afraid of. I don't want to remember that you never noticed my silence, my tears. Mommy, I don't want to remember that I told you — and you did nothing. Mommy, you told me no one would ever love me as much as my family. That scares me, Mommy. I don't want to be loved like that.

I wanted to be loved. I want to have fun. I don't want to be a child anymore; I don't want to be their victim, their survivor. I want to grow up. I don't want to fight the need to cut myself. I don't want to force myself to leave the house. I don't want to decide to live or die. I don't want to have to hurt myself because of old anger. I want it all to go away. I'm tired now, I want to sleep without your hands coming down on my body. I want a break. I want you to take it all away from me, Mommy — give it back to them. I want you all to feel bad so I can go out and play.

Deborah Lynn

A PROGRESS REPORT ON DEBORAH LYNN

Since I first wrote this piece, I've grown up and moved beyond the abuse that controlled much of my life and actions. This last summer, I completed more than ten years of therapy. Alyce and I had a wonderful dinner to celebrate! As I used to believe I was destined to live in a fog forever or to die, that night was very significant for me.

Critical to my recovery was reliving and accepting some of the feelings I experienced as a child. Facing those fears and the depth of my abuse was the most painful thing I have faced as an adult. I learned through this process, that healing was my responsibility, even though the abuse was never my fault. I worked like hell for that healing and I feel grateful that there can be so many good days in my life.

I now manage a farm with my partner and am also direct services coordinator for a rape crisis center in Southern California. It has been a long-time goal of mine to be strong enough and capable enough to give something back to the community that supported me so well during my healing and growing.

FIRST WE CREATE THE NIGHTMARES, THEN WE CREATE THE PRISONS

That afternoon as Susan began to read aloud, she cried after almost every sentence. Her wavy, long, red hair tumbled down her face as she bent her head to read, and several times she stopped and said, "I can't go on." The supportive silence of everyone in the room formed a safety net under her very young and yet very old small feet. She told her story of how at twelve she was raped and beaten by the houseboy while her wealthy father and professional mother worked. She was sent to a school for unwed mothers for nine months and then gave the baby up for adoption.

"Maybe I've had my ten kids after that because I always wanted to make up for that loss. I wanted to keep the baby but my mother said, 'No, it'll kill your father.' I mailed him letters from Canada where I was supposed to be but he never knew I was here in the states all the time. He still doesn't know to this day."

She laughed and cried at the same time. Tears streamed down her pale white skin. Someone handed her a toilet tissue roll and she looked up to smile "thank you" and broke into tears again.

Through the body of writing created over the past six years by the women inmates in the Bright Fires Creative Writing Program at California Rehabilitation Center, CRC (a medium-security prison, initially designed for people with problems of drug abuse, addiction, and drug-related crimes), I have learned about the re-lationship between child abuse and the incarceration of women.

In 1979, when I began at CRC, I had no idea that at least 90 percent of the women I worked with were victims of child abuse. Nor was I aware that at least 75 percent were victims of childhood sexual abuse.

Child abuse, because it so often leads to self-abuse, has played a major role in the lives of women at CRC. Self-abuse in adulthood may take the form of drug addiction, suicide, mental illness, and/ or crime. Thus, child abuse is an integral part of the road to prison for most women with whom I have worked.

A composite of many creative forces was working in the Bright Fires Writing Program at the beginning of 1983. For the first time in their lives, the women involved felt free and safe enough in a group (albeit in prison), to say out loud those words that had been forbidden them in the past. Until now, the taboo of speaking out this demon was too strong. They had been forbidden their voice until finally they didn't know they had one.

The following is a collection of writings from some of these women:

WAR STORIES

Women sharing
　　war stories
　　　　that can
　　　　　　only be told here
　　　　　　　　behind bars from
　　　　　　　　　　Middle America

War stories
　　of prostitution
　　　　nights in labor camps
　　　　　　not remembering
　　　　　　　　how many came

War stories
　　about the pain of addiction
　　　　kicking drugs
　　　　　　after three years running

War stories
　　of unwanted abortions
　　　　rapes of children
　　　　　　that grew to be
　　　　　　　　these women

Ryvonne L.

A LITTLE GIRL'S QUESTION

She wraps her arms
Tightly around herself
Rocking
Back and forth
Back and forth
Her mind lingers
Tears in her eyes
She can't remember
If daddy came home
But she hears a voice
deep
gruff
"C-mere, honey, sit on Daddy's lap,"
She bounces high
On a sturdy knee
laughing
until the pain
slid up her thigh
"Such a nice little girl,"
Came the sigh . . .

She wraps her arms
Tightly around herself
Rocking
Back and forth
Back and forth
Tears in her eyes
She still can't remember
If Daddy came home . . .

Sandy S.

Silent Rage

My mother died when I was only five days old. Although a very hard task lay ahead for him, my father took the burden of raising me, a girl, all alone.

He knew he couldn't continue without some kind of help, so he hired me out, as he would say, to people who didn't have children of their own.

I guess my father must have felt bad about leaving me with strangers, and one evening he drove up to the house in his big shiny black Oldsmobile and brought me a beautiful teddy bear.

My father told me he was giving Ted E. to me so he could watch out for me while he was away working. I loved Ted E. very much, and told him all of my secrets. We would play for hours, but I wouldn't lay him down because he was not washable.

One fall day I was sitting out on the back porch with Ted E. and squeezing him around the neck very hard, and his head fell off. I ran in the house yelling for someone to "fix him, fix him." Mr. Akright told me he would fix him, and took me by the hand and led me down the cellar stairs where the furnace was blazing and opened the furnace door. He then took the head of my faithful companion and grabbed me by my hair and, holding my head back, he told me to watch as he threw Ted E.'s head into the flames. I tried to run away from him because I thought he would also throw me in after him. But he held me fast and laughed. This I believe was the first time in my life I ever felt hate.

That night, after I was put to bed, I still felt the rage in my heart. After the door was closed, I took a fist full of my crayolas and completely covered every inch of walls and furnishings that were in my reach. After I had exhausted myself, I climbed back into the crib and fell fast asleep. I was awakened the next morning by the ranting and raving of Mrs. Akright who was saying how she didn't want such a horrid little girl under her roof. She called my father and when he arrived told him that I was a vicious little girl whom no one would take care of for long.

When we got out to the car, my father told me if I always told him the truth that he would be on my side. When I explained to him why I felt I had to do what I did, he was very understanding. He didn't spank me, but he told me I should have told him and he would have handled it in another way. He did see my side and knew how I must have felt. A few months after this happened they committed Mr. Akright to a mental home where he passed away. To this day I always feel it is better to tell the truth no matter how bad things seem to be.

Pat

Did He Really

"You're no good,"
Aunt Lora would say,

> As young arms would strive
> to shield the young girl from
> blows from the massive woman
>
>> "You're good,"
>> Uncle Homer said.

"You're evil-minded,"
Aunt Lora would say

> When the child would
> ask some naive question
> about something she'd
> heard in school
>
>> "It's only natural
>> to ask,"
>> Uncle Homer would
>> whisper in hushed
>> tones.

"Until you see the light,"
Aunt Lora would shout

> Slamming the old shed door
> sometimes for days
>
>> "I brought you
>> something to eat."
>> Uncle Homer would
>> say much later.

"I saw you talking to that new boy
today, you little tramp,"
Aunt Lora would hiss
                    Driving home
                    the child cringing
                    expecting another blow
                                        "Boys ain't all
                                        bad," Uncle Homer
                                        would say.

"Don't expect to hug me,
I don't like to be touched,"
Aunt Lora would pull away
                    from any affection
                    the child had to offer
                                        Uncle Homer loved
                                        hugs and kisses.

"Go to the chicken coop and stay,"
Aunt Lora would scream
                    as company of
                    brothers, cousins and others
                    would come on Sunday visits
                                        "Wanna go fishing?"
                                        Uncle Homer would
                                        retrieve
                                        her from her
                                        feathered
                                        prison.

"No one wants you,"
Aunt Lora would bellow
                    as the young girl would
                    walk into the living room
                                        "I want you,"
                                        Uncle Homer would
                                        say in
                                        his slow Southern
                                        drawl.

"No one loves you,"
Aunt Lora would insist
                when the girl would
                ask about her
                mother and brother
                                "I love you,"
                                Uncle Homer would
                                say
                                as he gently
                                pulled down
                                her white cotton
                                panties.

                                        Ryvonne L.

WILL THE REAL CRIMINAL PLEASE STAND UP

She was six
He was thirty

She was a child with raven hair
and ivory skin

Fragile innocence
a young princess like you'd meet
in Brothers Grimm

     Except

he caught her
held back her flailing arms,
tore at her party dress
inserted pain

For years she lived in paralysis
afraid for anyone to touch her
she imagined spiders
and other crawling things
living inside her

at eight

    at nine

      at ten

again and again
she cried Momma, Momma,
He whispered, "I'll kill you if you tell."

till one day she found him
with her sister
she told her Grandma
who hit him on the head with a frying pan
till he grew into a monster
and threw the ninety-year-old woman out the window

    she died soon after

the little girl escaped
years later she found PCP
her drug of choice to kill the pain

married
    frigid
      insane
        and Norman?

      He is still free.

Sharon S.

FINDING A VOICE

The taboo against speaking about child abuse, especially sexual abuse, has been so great that the victims have lost their own voices. They have been told "Don't tell or I'll kill." They have been forced to swallow their own voices and thus to lose or negate an essential part of themselves.

As a result I came to understand my role very clearly in this prison. There was a great need to discover this lost, forgotten or hidden voice. The gift of creative writing became the tool for this exploration and communication. We learned to talk to each other in writing, to break the silence, to tell secrets.

The expiation of repressed guilt, blame, rage, and sorrow after so many years was critical for any growth or change. People need the mourning and a compassionate listener. They need rituals for imaginative confrontations with their fear of speaking out, or a workshop setting which allows them to release their own voice, thereby releasing the voices of others. The whole atmosphere of repression is lifted.

The notion of the voice, the ability to express all the feelings and emotions that have been repressed due to this childhood trauma, is the important key here. It has been with the lifting of the voice through the creation of a work of art in the form of prose, poetry, or dramatic dialogue and the subsequent presentation of this art form to the larger public that has served to free many of the women with whom I have worked. These were points of transformation. No one was ever the same after this. Many who went through this process are on their way to healing.

Sharon Sticker, Director
Bright Fires Creative Writing Program
California Rehabilitation Center

I WILL NOT

No.

I will not allow it.

I know who you are and I name you.

I know what you want and I will not do it.

I will not let the forces of your death impinge upon my life.

No more.

I will not let myself only survive.

I will not let myself slowly die of uncare, lack of care.

You convinced me that no one cared but I no longer believe you

I will not isolate myself in my pain.

You did that.

I will not hurt myself, put myself down, cut myself, tie myself
    up, touch myself wrongly or violently, put things into my body
    that do not belong there.

I will not do any of the things you did to me.

I will not do any of the things you made me do, or made me
    think I could do, or think I did, and still want from me.

I will not sexually abuse.

I will not hate. I will not even be cynical.

I will not kill, myself or anyone or anything else.

I will not hurt babies or children or animals.

I will not project your evil into animals.

I will never again sit back and watch atrocities without
    feeling. I will feel.

I am not evil like you, like you tried to tell me I am.

I am not the stupid idiot you tried to scream into existence.

I have feelings, though you tried to take them away, and then
    used the empty space for your atrocities, your fun, evil laughter.

But I am not fooled.

It was not me.

I am not you. I am not your evil.

And I will not allow it within me anymore.

I will not rage with such chaos that my loved ones leave me.

I will not rage at my own children. I will not hurt them with
    your abusive hands or voices or hearts.

I will keep them in the light and give them freedom.
Yes, I rage. But I rage vitality.
I am full of vitality, full of life and life-giving force.
I am full of goodness, of God, of Jesus, of Great Spirit,
    full of real power and real gentleness.
And I will not let you continue.
I will never again let your death be in me.
I rage life. I breathe love. I offer Peace.
And I do not allow you.
BE GONE
Let my innocence and my purity be enough to frighten you into
nothing.

Anonymous

RAW INTELLECT

My father was a simple man
A simpleton
Raised without means

Lacking of education
Desiring only to exist.

I do not follow in his footsteps.
The son meant to stride
The daughters, to crawl in the dust.

I crave knowledge
Shining golden fleece
Even that I can't grasp.

I muse that all in life is fairer with knowledge.

How selfish I have become
Prostituting my self-esteem.

Remember those words?
We can only afford to send one of you to college.

Using others for their intellect

Like a vulture.

I descend wherever the talk is the thickest.

N.V. Bennett

MR. WIZARD

At night the shadows creep into my room.
I pretend to sleep.
They prod me awake with their iron staffs.

They have seen me cry.
Pillow forced hard on child's jaw.
They keep on coming, although I wish them away.

There's a giant lurking at my morning table.
Daddy says, "Did you sleep well princess?"

N.V. Bennett

A PROGRESS REPORT ON N.V. BENNETT

I live happily on Vancouver Island with my second husband and my two daughters. My personal cycle of abuse, which began at age five, ended when I left my first husband several years ago. I have found writing for me the best way to work out my anger and my fear. I have achieved the ability to accept my own importance and intelligence. With the help of my new husband I am determined to raise our daughters to have pride in who they are and to believe in all they can attain.

MOVING BEYOND THE DARKNESS:
Insights And Perceptions

Stepping into the light is an experience all survivors long for. Along the continuum of healing, the light becomes brighter the longer and harder you strive for recovery. Clients tell me that when they move to the place in their recovery that is beyond the darkness, they realize that there really is more to life than just surviving. In my practice, I collect fairy godmother magic wands. I wish I had a magic wand to take away your hurt and make everything better, but, alas, there is no magic to be found in this process. This is a journey that lasts a lifetime. Rest assured that each stage of the struggle will make you a stronger person.

While you cannot ever change or erase what happened in your past, I believe that you have the power to choose what you do with what happened. Recovery is reclaiming your abusive past, recognizing that it is a part of your life's history and identity, feeling the loss and grief of the past and finally, letting go of the trauma. Once you deal with your emotions, you can begin to integrate them into your life. This integration process does not mean that you no longer remember the past or cease to feel the feelings associated with it, instead you are freed to remember and to feel. Start now to rewrite the outcome of your life's story.

The experiences, the visions, and the effects of your abuse will fade away but not completely. There will always be faded memories, but know that recovery is really possible. As you gather in the healing light, you will be victorious and triumph over darkness.

Wendy Ann Wood

CHAPTER FOUR

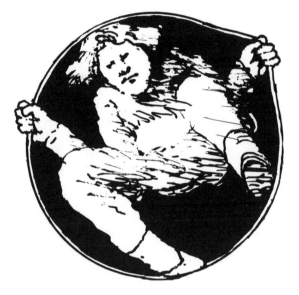

VOICES OF RITUAL
ABUSE SURVIVORS

MYTHS AND FACTS ABOUT RITUAL ABUSE

Myth: *Ritual abuse in day care settings rarely, if ever, occurs.*
Fact: According to a recently completed study by the federal government, ritual abuse and child molestation occurs in up to 20 percent of day care centers. Parents need to continue to exercise basic precautions in selecting any caretakers for their children.

Myth: *Just look at the bizarre stories that have been occurring in the media lately; of course, they are untrue.*
Fact: What is bizarre to one culture is commonplace to another. Offenders often add bizarre features to abuses to make the crime seem unbelievable.

Myth: *Survivors will not be believed. They will just create hell for themselves and their families by going public. The "bad guys" are stronger than everyone else. Don't trust anyone.*
Fact: Sometimes the effort to stop the "bad guy" does not work, but you know you tried. Often speaking out encourages other victims who also need help to come forward. Some people do not believe the survivor. However, there is a growing number of people who believe and are willing to help survivors place blame where it is due — on the offender. Keep telling until you are heard.

Myth: *As a therapist, cases of child ritual abuse are a sure way to involve yourself in very stressful legal battles.*
Fact: The legal system can never legitimately ask a therapist to be a fact finder for the court. The therapist, as a private care provider for the client, also enjoys client confidentiality under the law in most cases.

Myth: *Ritual abuse cases involving children are a "no win" for everyone, and a "no file" decision as far as criminal charges are concerned.*
Fact: Superior Court Judge William Pounders has remarked that the McMartain Preschool case has "poisoned" the lives of everyone it has touched. Without remedies, this case will also poison the lives of those in similar cases.

Myth: *These social and criminal problems are too hot to touch. Any legislative proposal offends either the civil libertarians or victim advocates or law enforcement — it costs too much anyway.*
Fact: To do nothing is even more costly. To leave the general public so dissatisfied with the process will discourage adults from going to authorities or therapists with their concerns about child abuse, leaving children unprotected and without therapy.

Statistics On Ritual Abuse

As the awareness of ritual abuse increases, professionals will begin to conduct more and more research on the actual statistics pertaining to the crime. Currently, law enforcement combines ritual crimes with sexual abuse statistics. This must change before we can fully understand the scope of ritual abuse. Professionals need to become aware of and recognize the reality of ritual abuse, before the true work can begin. Hopefully, it will only be a matter of time until we can address the many unanswered questions on the subject of ritual abuse.

- In a study on "Multi-generational Satanic Cult Involvement" by Driscoll and Wright done in 1991, 93 percent of ritual abuse survivors were found to be female.

- 84 percent of survivors studied reported human sacrifice was involved in their abuse (Driscoll and Wright, 1991).

- According to Driscoll and Wright, females comprised 25 percent of the reported perpetrators.

- 76 percent of survivors reported that child pornography occurred as part of cult abuse (Cook, 1991).

- 25 percent of all clients diagnosed with multiple personality disorder (MPD) are survivors of childhood ritual abuse (Braun, 1989).

- 79 percent of survivors said that Christianity was either "perverted or inverted" during rituals (Cook, 1991).

A WORD OF CAUTION

I want to caution you that the material in this chapter may be extremely upsetting. I urge you to follow your own judgment and instinct in deciding whether to read this material or not. Use extreme caution if you are in the early stages of working on your own ritual abuse memories. It is important to keep your memories clear and uncontaminated, until you can begin to process them with a therapist. Reading this might cause you confusion, misunderstanding, disbelief and/or denial, and perhaps increase your fear of the recovery process. What ever you decide to do, take care of yourself first and foremost.

Because these writings are extremely powerful, violent, and graphic, I have taken the liberty (with the authors' permission) to omit some of the most gruesome experiences. I feel that you can grasp the impact and intensity of the abuse from the remaining material.

I realize that this chapter may be overwhelming and difficult to read, but I also want to emphasize that this type of abuse does happen. If child abuse is going to stop, we must give society a reason to stop it. Even though the material may make many readers uncomfortable, we cannot turn the tragedy of abuse into a fairy tale. The hopeful endings depicted throughout come from determination, hard work, and the guts to come forward and survive the ordeal. I hope these stories make a difference.

Playing By The "Rules"

Voices in the background, chanting, chanting . . .
　　play by the "rules" or you are out
　　the "rules" change from game to game,
　　　' from play to play, from minute to minute

The "rules" govern
　　the "rules" are everything
　　　　the "rules" determine who stays, who goes
　　　　who is loved, who is ignored
　　　　who is rewarded, who is punished

The "rules" are complicated, intricate
　　determined by the rule giver
　　who determines the punishment, the penalty

The "rules" are traps, waiting to snag, waiting to catch,
　　waiting to kill . . .
　　　　. . . kill the spirit
　　　　. . . kill the soul
　　　　. . . kill the fire within

When I was little, I was governed by the "rules"
　　I tried to play by the "rules"
　　I tried to interpret the "rules"

And part of me died . . .

Diane

DONE TO YOU

Done to you
Done to you
Many things were
Done to you
They were dirty
They were bad
All those things they
Did to you.
You held on
And went along
With all those things they
Did to you.
But you had no idea to run away
There was no place to safely play
Those black marks on your soul would stay
If you dared a word to say.
A bad, bad girl, you'd burn someday
If you fought those things that were
Done to you.

Rylee B.

WARPED ALLIANCES

My life
Has been filled
With
Warped alliances
Obsessions about
Your reactions, your needs,
Your feelings, your wants,
Your perceptions, your desires.
Not that it is
Wrong
To care
For you
But it is
Deadly
To care less
For
Me.
See
What
I
Mean?
Warped Alliances.

Rylee B.

A PROGRESS REPORT ON RYLEE

"Rylee B." is the pseudonym used by this thirty-six-year-old survivor of sexual and ritualistic abuse. In 1986, explaining years of illness and puzzling symptoms, she was diagnosed as having a multiple personality disorder, stemming from the trauma of her abuses.

For the past three years Rylee has worked closely with a psychologist, and together they have uncovered the secrets that have tormented her for so long. In seeing and understanding the basis for her illness, Rylee and her psychologist are beginning to reach and heal her many personalities.

Writing in journals, composing poetry, and music, rekindling a relationship with God, and meeting and developing relationships with other abuse survivors helps Rylee in her daily struggle to overcome her early traumas. Rylee lives in Oregon with her husband and four children.

JEANNE'S STORY

I am a thirty-nine-year-old female and I am just at the beginning of unearthing the memories of the ritual abuse to which I was subjected. Prior to November, 1989, I had very few memories of my childhood from birth to age thirteen. With the help and protection of a gifted, loving therapist I began to get memories of having been incested by my mother, father and both my brothers. I am slowly recovering from those experiences and continue to go to therapy five times a week, attend two sessions weekly of Incest Survivor's Anonymous (ISA), and am taking counseling classes which support my personal growth. Having built-in support systems that are an ongoing part of my daily life is crucial to my recovery.

As is the experience of most incest survivors, recalling memories is both excruciatingly painful and tremendously relieving. At last pieces of my life begin to make sense to me. But at an even deeper level, I know there must be more. Even the sadistic nature and the constantness of the incest of which I was a victim from infancy to at least age seven (I still have no memory from age seven to thirteen) did not explain the depth of my pain or self-contempt. I knew there must be more.

In the ISA meetings I attended there is one woman who is also an incest and ritual abuse survivor. At the first meeting I attended in which she was present, I was immediately drawn to her. She has since told me that she knew as soon as I walked in the room that I was a ritual abuse survivor. I listened intently every time she talked. At the close of that first meeting, she came across the room and held my hand as we said the closing prayer. I looked at her and said, "You understand, don't you?" She said, "Yes."

Shortly thereafter I got my first memory of what I believe was part of the ritual abuse. I was seven years old and was told to sit outside the door of the middle bedroom in my mother's house while my mother and at least two other adults were in that room performing some sort of activity. The door opens and I am told to come in. I know that they want something from me and then I will be allowed to leave. They want my urine. They lay me on either a bed or table, put a dish under me and make me pee in it. To this day, I am terrified of using a bed pan.

In my next memory I am four or five years old. I am in that same bedroom in my mother's house. My mother is there, as are two or three other adults and a young boy. My clothes are removed and I am instructed to spread my legs apart and just lie still. My mother is yelling at me to shut up and just lie there. They are telling me that I am evil and that this is Jesus who is entering his penis into my body and that they are trying to save me. The boy is scared too, and at first I sense that he does not want to do this. But then he seems to start getting enjoyment from it and I begin to hate him too.

When I was three or four years old my father made me lie down on a table and held me down while my mother forced a cross all the way into my vagina. I remember the pain as the horizontal bar on the cross was forced into me and I remember my father yelling to my mother, "Do it!" I do not remember much else from that experience except that it seems they thought they were trying to rid me of some sort of evil.

Also at the age of two and three, my mother and father would sit me in a chair in the kitchen and tie down my legs and right arm. My mother would hold my left arm while my father would cut my wrist with a sharp knife. I would then have to stand at the table and let my blood drip into a jar. I do not know what they did with the blood. After having this memory I came home and told my husband about it. He looked at my wrist and saw tiny scars left by my father's knife. The scars are reassuring in that they validate my memory, and terrifying because they do not let me deny the experience.

To keep me from telling anyone what was going on in my mother's home (I do not call it my home), my mother would fill the bath tub with scalding hot water. Beginning at the age of two, and possibly before, she would begin by dipping me into the water while singing:

"Put the baby in the water.
Watch the baby burn.
Teach this baby not to tell.
This is how she'll learn.
Bad Baby. Bad, Bad Baby!"

She would then hold me completely under the water for what seemed like a few minutes. I remember wishing there were a handle on the bottom of the bath tub that I could hold on to so that I would never have to come up and face her again.

My recovery

I know there is still a lot more that I have to remember and re-experience. I am trying to be patient and compassionate with myself and trust my process. I keep telling myself that since I got through the original trauma, I can get through the memories. They seem to come in clusters of three. I have not had a new one in almost five days now and I find myself anxious about when the next one will come. I want them back because I want to reclaim my childhood and make sense of my life. Yet I am terrified of them. Each time I remember, it is as if the experience is happening all over again. Except this time, I am not going through it alone. I have my therapist who is there with me and I have people I can tell. I do not have to keep it a secret any longer and that is healing. I do not know the context in which the ritual abuse was performed; I imagine I will someday. Right now, that does not seem too important. What seems important is finding that small child inside me who went into hiding thirty-nine years ago and who needs to tell her story, experience her pain, fear and rage, and learn that she is a beautiful, precious little girl who deserves to be welcomed into the world.

Jeanne P.

A PROGRESS REPORT ON JEANNE

I can not yet honestly say that I am happy but I believe, for the first time in my life, that happiness is attainable. Before I remembered the abuse, I had always thought I was born to be unhappy. Sometimes I thought I was crazy. I am not. They did not win and they did not reach my center — and they never will. I survived the abuse and now I am learning to live.

KAREN'S STORY

Sometimes when I am feeling real bad, a song comes floating into my head. I have noticed generally, as a rule, the song has great significance as to what I am feeling or remembering at that moment. I know as a child I zeroed in on music as an escape from the trauma of existing in a home with crazy alcoholic parents. Music carried me. Gave me softness in a harsh world. Gave me dreams of one day being rescued by a person who would love me and want me. It is no wonder I am particularly partial to '50s and '60s music. I was a small child in the '50s and on into puberty in the '60s. Those are the years I have very little recollection of. The forgotten years I thought everyone never remembered. Now, since I have been in recovery, I keep remembering. The memories come as great punches in the gut, severe headaches, unbelievable female cramps, eyes wanting to cry but frozen, constant flu and exhaustion, periods of complete disorientation, hurting all over. Then I want to punch myself, I scream at assholes, and I can't sleep at night. There are times when I think I cannot bear it another hour or another day, days when people all seem cruel, foreign and out to harm me.

I had a stepfather who was a psychopath. He liked to fuck women and kill them in the act. And if that wasn't enough, he enjoyed dragging his five-year-old stepdaughter along with him and forced her to watch. He made her stab them too to make her believe that she was responsible. He and my mother made money off that child with pornography. She was made to participate in orgies and Satanic rituals. The entire group once peed and shit on her. The horrors are endless. She was beaten all her life. It never ended. She even grew up to find a husband to beat her.

And then my therapist informs me to expect at least three more years of flooding ritual memories. It feels like a judge giving me a jail sentence. Okay, you were unfortunate enough to be born to a very sick mother; therefore, the punishment is a lifetime of either acting out a childhood hell or remembering a childhood hell. Who is in control? The twelve-step groups tell me my Higher Power. He has sentenced me to recovery. Which spells PAIN. It is not always this bad. Sometimes life is full of love and support. But I forget. Most times I forget. I was brainwashed so well. So very well. Brainwashed by those sick evil people. Led to believe that no one would help. No one would want to help. I am unworthy of help. I am sickening if I turn for help. I'll be punished. I can't be weak or I'll be punished. I am to suffer. And sometimes I believe, if I pretend, it is not happening and it will all go away.

The song I keep hearing today is, "Come back when you grow up, girl/ You're still living in a paper doll world/ Living ain't easy, loving's twice as tough/ So come back, baby, when you grow up." Then Janis Joplin kicks in with, "Hold on, just a little bit tighter now, baby." I can't give up now. They would win. No way will I let them win!

Karen G.

A PROGRESS REPORT ON KAREN

I have come a long way. I was once in a tiny fantasy world, angry, furious, and pissed off. Sleeping with men I picked up in bars. Relocating every six months to a year. Living in a constant drug-induced zombie land. Now I am responsible. I no longer hang out with men who beat me. I have been clean and sober for four years now. I have my degree. I have friends who are healthy. I go to an incest support group and have a fabulous therapist. I am spiritual. I have hope. I am learning a healthy lifestyle. I am a miracle! My son would be happy to confirm that for you. It is tough remembering the ritual abuse. I still need help, lots of help. That makes me sad sometimes, but maybe I will learn that I am lovable in the process. I sure hope so.

SILENT INSANITY

You threatened me with wild eyes, shaking fingers.
You threatened me to never speak a word.
And screams and blood and death and darkness,
Like a hurricane in my three-year-old head,
Blew around and around and deep, deep down,
Condemning me to silent insanity.

Frantic screams from wide mouth fiends
Told me to promise and swear out to all,
Reminding me that I was a daughter
To one and to all and to the Devil himself.
But fear clamped my mouth shut
And fear took my breath;
So I spoke not a word, I swore not a word.
And the hurricane blew in my three-year-old head,
Around and around and deep, deep down,
Condemning me to silent insanity.

So you carried me off like a pig to the slaughter;
You carried me off to a region of hell
Where fire is icy freezing but it burns all the same.
You placed me among little daughters of Satan
Slaughtered then frozen in this region of hell,
And you left me to sit with my hurricane blowing
Around and around and deep, deep down,
Condemning me to silent insanity.

As my bones shook in coldness, but more so in fear,
I swore and I swore and I swore once again.
And just as death was about to release me from bondage,
You opened the door that led back to life —
Life with the darkness, life with the blood,
Life with the hurricane in my three-year-old head,
And it blew and it blew now deep down inside me,
Condemning me to silent insanity.

Linda M.

Tell What?

Mama said:
Don't tell you evil child!

Daddy said:
Don't tell you dirty bitch!

Gordon said:
Don't tell or I will hurt you!

Danny said:
Don't tell because I love you!

They all said:
No one will believe you!

And in time I said:
Who cares anyway?

Because, I said when I was six
And her Mama wouldn't
Let her play with me again.

Because, I said when I was ten
And she believed but no one else cared
They made me say I lied.

Because, I said when I was fifteen
And there was HELL to pay.

By then
It was not Mama
It was not Daddy
It was not Gordon
It was not Danny
Who said:

DON'T TELL!
It was Satan,
And I lived in hell.

Then I learned that telling
Meant pain, not for me
But for someone else,
And I had to watch and know
They hurt because I told.

And even if
I thought of telling
I paid.
They knew.
They always knew.
And one day I stopped thinking.
But every night
I heard them say:
DON'T TELL!
And I said:
Tell what?

Linda M.

METAMORPHOSIS

Child in Darkness
Woman in Light
Nature worked Her miracle.
From crawly thing
To great winged beauty
Nature worked her miracle.

And now I soar
Far above the dark,
Dreaded world
And now I am free
As Nature meant for me to be.
And I rejoice
With a heart of love
Nature's birthing gift to me.

And I hear whispers
"Metamorphosis"
Out of caves and into canyons
Until I hear it thundering
"Metamorphosis!!"

Quill in one hand
A mighty sword of justice
in the other
And a voice that is mine
To shout around the world.

Bloody bits of shadowy slivers
Once razor sharp, now dulled
Lie broken.
Silence is no more.

And I hear whispers
"Metamorphosis"
From those yet to feel
Her transformation.
But they believe
Because they see me.

Child of Darkness
Woman of Light
Nature worked her miracle —
Metamorphosis!

Linda M.

DEAR LINDA, DEAREST LINDA
(A Letter To Myself)

Dear Linda,

Will you be my friend?

The pain I can numb; the rage I can hide away; but the loneliness consumes me. This feeling of abandonment eats away my soul like cancer. I tire of being the only one to wipe my tears away, to hug my shaking body. I have this desire to feel the warmth of a loving embrace, a supportive embrace is causing me a grief too strong to endure. When I sit in my room, four dull walls surround me and all I hear are the echoes of my sobs. I pray for a caring voice to tell me she understands, believes and loves me. For four months I talked to a little friend that could be my very own. And we grew close and our hearts became one. I died inside and out when I had to turn my little one over to the care of, hopefully, a caring God. I knew, however, that first he would have to pass through the pains of Hell. I feel so utterly alone. I can no longer dry my tears or hug my shaking body.

Please, please will you be my friend?

Linda
Age 15

Dearest Linda,

I want to always be your friend. I understand, I believe, and I love you.

You will always have a friend!

Linda
Age 36

Linda M.

A PROGRESS REPORT ON LINDA

I have been in therapy for three years now and my recovery from incest is remarkable considering where I was when I entered treatment. My greatest desire as a warrior now is to have my poetry and writings published. This, to me, is the ultimate victory over my abusers.

I still have much work to do on all of my abuse issues. But as I look back on the last three years since I have been in treatment, I recognize the immense progress I have made and continue to make. The key to my recovery is found in one statement: "I am not alone anymore!"

UNANSWERED QUESTIONS . . . ANSWERED!

All of my life I felt incomplete, that there had to be more to me then meets the eye. I had many strange sensations about death; part of me wanted to die and I could not explain it. I also had a lot of phobias about blood, snakes, needles, sick people, heights and electricity. But I always thought that phobias were just part of a normal life. Then there was the anger. This anger was extremely intense. I had many outbursts for apparently no reason. This anger was what my family and friends complained about the most.

When I thought of my mother I wanted to kill her. I always knew that she was evil, but I never knew how evil until she died. She died of pneumonia in a foster home. My husband and I went to see her often, not for her but for me. She put me through hell all of my life and I did not want to feel guilty when she died. When she did die I finally felt free, but not free enough, something was still missing.

One day I made an emergency appointment with my therapist and she suggested we go about finding and knowing my roots. That day changed my life. Going back I remember being three years old and my mother smothered my baby sister while she thought I was asleep. That was my first sense of loss and the beginning of many horrible things that happened to me. After divorcing my father (he knew nothing of this) we moved into a house where I began to be ritualistically abused.

I would go to sleep and wake up with people in robes around my bed. My mother would be drawing blood or trying to take a urine sample from me. Once I awoke with snakes crawling on my naked body. People took pictures of me, I was beaten and sexually abused. Never was I loved and rarely was I fed or bathed. I was just a sad-eyed zombie given drugs to keep me quiet and calm.

As of yet it is unclear how long this went on but I now realize why I had so many problems in my life. So many unanswered questions got answers. Now I feel like a person, finally I feel whole. The nightmare of my past still haunts me but I am so thankful that I did not become like my mother. I am so thankful for my friends, my family, my husband and God.

Marylin

THE WARM DARK SMELLY SLIME

I feel like a queen dressed in the very best!
With beauty inside and out.

Everything neat, and just right
Beautiful jewels of diamonds and pearls
Rose lace on a white satin dress.
Upon my head, a crown with the most fragrant flowers.

I walk through a field of colorful flowers.
Everywhere, there are soaring birds and fluttering butterflies.
The new day sun shines brightly upon my face and the
Beauty of nature surrounds me in peacefulness.

Suddenly, I feel something, and warm dark smelly slime
Has fallen from the sky upon my face that once shined with
     the glow of the sun.

Now covered in darkness,
No longer a smile, but a face of fear.
No longer the smell of the freshness of life. I gasp,
As I am smothered by the warm dark smelly slime.

I can't stand it!
I must find my way out from under this pile
Deeper and thicker than I could ever image, I
Become hidden by the warm dark smelly slime.

I wade through, stopping from time to time
Gasping for air. I gain some energy to dig once more
Through the warm dark smelly slime.

I picture in my mind a field of the most fragrant flowers,
Soaring birds, fluttering butterflies and a new day sun shining
     against my face.

I am frightened, then angry, angry then frightened.
I must find water and fresh smelling soap to wash away
The filth of the warm dark smelly slime.

The journey seems long with no end in sight.
Sometimes discouraged and in deep despair
I feel I will never reach the end of the
Warm dark smelly slime.

Muffled in the distance, I think I hear the sound
Of a babbling brook. My vision is blurred and I strain
To hear and see what lies before me
Through the warm dark smelly slime.

I keep moving on, one foot in front of the other.
I am drawn by a force to reach what sounds like crystal clear
     water.
I pause, and wipe away from my eyes, ears and mouth,
The warm dark smelly slime.

The sound gets clearer. My eyes can begin to see.
Is it true? Am I right? Finally, overwhelmed with
Excitement, strength and energy I realize it is true, a brook
At last to wash what is left of the warm dark smelly slime.

I reach the water's edge and I plunge in with force.
It is cold, refreshing and a relief. Washing as fast as I can
I begin to realize that it does not come off as fast as I
Would like, the warm dark smelly slime.

I begin to see soaring birds, fluttering butterflies and smell
The most fragrant flowers. I feel the warmth of the new
Day sun shining brightly on my face.
Oh yes, the sound of the babbling brook that washed
Away the warm dark smelly slime.

I will always have memories of the darkness, the smell,
The feel, the muffle, and the stain on my dress to remind me.
But, there is a breath of life, I can raise my head high,
I am no longer buried by the warm dark smelly slime.

Patrice F.

A PROGRESS REPORT ON PATRICE

I have just completed one year of recovery from sexual abuse.
Sometimes it is hard to remember why I ever began, but then I
realize just how far I have come. For me the turning point in my
life came when I began to take my recovery one day at a time and
when I realized that I may continue to work on these issues for the
rest of my life. I find it encouraging and healing to help those who
are just beginning their recovery journey. We are pioneers in a new
and greater understanding of sexual abuse. We are the ones who
can make a difference and make the changes so that generations
to come may have greater peace and more functional lives.

CODE OF SILENCE, CODE OF DEATH

Skip lightly, skip lightly my child,
Stern injunction of eggshell'd silence
In fierce squinty eyes —
No words needed.

Speak tightly, speak tightly my child.
Bridge of lies built by lisping lips
Between reality and life —
Heart's tomb concealed.

Look brightly, look brightly my child,
Glaring scintillation off broken glass
Blinds to truth of emptiness —
Clowning deception believed.

She walked lightly, spoke tightly, looked brightly
To save her skin from death's most tortuous knell,
That heart's hidden grave undiscovered would remain —
But such a life to live is worse than hell.

She believed his gambit-string words,
That she'd keep her candle lit
By giving up her soul to him,
By dying bit by bit.

He used deception's mask to fool
For self-besotted whim
Till none remained of childish life
Save shell of light most dim.

Sarah K.

MY HIDDEN ROOM

The secret door to an unknown room
Deep within my soul has been exposed.
Curiosity strikes
So I crack it open just a bit —
And slam it shut in fear.
Full of all uncleanness it is,
And angry furniture dedicated
Toward hating the one
I'm supposed to love.

Who is this lovable hated one?
A wizened caricature of holiness
Sitting on a ricketed throne
Appears before my tainted eyes,
Who demands absolutely
Enslaved perfection,
Whose promising words
Crack apart before they leave his mouth.
Who keeps his thoughts of me
stacked beside him
Like so many porn-queen magazines,
Ready for him to flip through,
      Ogle over,
            And act on.

Thoughts of terror engulf me
And I seek in futile wonder to hide
From this All-knowing one
With the penetrating madness
A burning fire in his eyes and hands,
Shaking out through his body
To ensnare and destroy me.

Is this the God I am supposed to know
And love?

Or is this a different god
Indelibly carved on my memory of stone
By design of evil
From a father who said he saw God,
   Knew God,
      And was God?

Who is the real True God?
How do I break apart the Rosetta Stone
Of the god of my childhood
To start afresh a clean tablet
Unperverted by the sacrificial knife
Defiled by blood of evil?
I do not know how to love this new God.
My pure gifts were spurned by the one
Who said he was God.

How can I love a God I do not know?
How can I trust a God of different memory
Or no memory?
How can I vow to serve this new God
When the old Rosetta law code is still extant
With no hope of destruction,
So that I know not how
To separate Old from New?

I fear to open the door
To this hidden room I have found.
Which god will lead me inside
To help me clean it out?

Sarah K.

A LETTER TO THE EDITOR

Editor's Note: The following letter was written to a major newspaper in Michigan and they could not [or would not] print it. I have included it here because we cannot keep silent any longer! The material may be too graphic for many readers. Please listen to your inner self when making your choice to read this material or not.

To the editor:

I am very concerned about the acquittal on the Buckley/McMartin case involving the sexual abuse of children in a California preschool. I had not been following the case because it has been too distressing to me. However, I could not stay in denial any longer after hearing and reading some of the reasons why the jurors did not find the McMartin/Buckleys guilty.

I understand that the jurors were "put off" by the "fantastic tales of animal mutilation, Satanic ritual and blood-letting," which seemed to taint even seemingly better documented cases (*The Ann Arbor News,* Friday, Jan. 19, 1990, p. A7).

I am concerned about the degree of denial in our society. Animal and human sacrifice can be used to sexually abuse children and keep them quiet about the abuse afterward. I should know. As a middle-aged professional woman with postgraduate degrees, the latest of which is from the University of Michigan, I lead a quiet life. I am very successful at my career and have earned the praise of employees, co-workers, and supervisors alike, most of whom are mental health professionals. I present a facade of competence and composure.

On the inside, I carry a living hell of memories which plague me day and night, especially night. Unfortunately, I am not psychotic, for then I would have some moments of relief. For you see, as a child from infancy to age six or seven, my parents were involved in "Satanic ritual" activities. You would not begin to believe the torture that I have experienced and witnessed. Like the children in California, my story changed over time because of my desire to deny the truth, the fact that I was sometimes drugged, and the desire to protect my caregivers, whom I, incidentally, loved despite what they did to me. For I was a child after all, and children are like that.

When one sees a cat splashed with a flammable liquid and set afire and then is told this is what will happen if s/he tells, the memory begins to wander. My own fuzzy details might not hold up in court where testimony had to be in a structure that interferes with the truth of the heart. The bottom line is that I was tortured and witnessed it in others. The bottom line is that this stuff does happen!

As a child actor in child pornography, I have experienced movies that reenact these horrors. There was a difference between cold chicken livers and animal blood and the temperature, texture and smell of human flesh and blood. Some of the details of the latter may be sometimes foggy and sometimes extremely vivid, but I have a cellular memory that will not quit. It is something that does not wash out with time and age.

Power and control: It is time that we begin to become aware of some individuals' and groups' desire for deviancy. Concentration camps are not only in history and on other continents. The children that I knew were tortured predominately in their own homes or those of their relatives. My mother attended Mass and communion daily. We were an attractive, middle class, good-looking family.

Sexual obsessions and perversions abounded forty years ago when I was a child. I imagine they still do today. The desire to use others for one's own gratification is not limited to California. Drugs weakened what little self-control my parents had. Those drugs and new, cheaper, fancier, and more powerful ones are even more prevalent today.

Nobody saw me, nobody listened then. My heart goes out to the children in California and their families who were brave enough to prosecute. I believe you. I do not know all the details, and you may not either. It does not matter. Something bad happened; something very bad. That is enough for me. Even if a court of law will not protect children, I will step forward and say I believe and I hope other grown-ups who have been through bad things will too. We need to start listening to the children. We need to start listening to our own truth.

Unfortunately, I cannot sign my name. I carry a victim's shame and publicity about this would be disruptive to my career.

Susan

SOME THOUGHTS FOR PROFESSIONALS WORKING WITH RITUALLY ABUSED SURVIVORS

This list is meant for professionals but may also be useful for survivors when seeking professional help on ritual abuse issues. Rephrase these suggestions into questions when you interview potential therapists. (More information on choosing a therapist can be found in *Resources*.)

1. **Develop your own personal boundaries prior to working with this clientele:** Before you start, know what you will and will not do when working with ritual abuse clients. Be flexible, but adhere strictly to your professional code of ethics. Beware of doing anything that promotes any type of "negative specialness" with the client.

2. **If you have a faint heart, avoid working with ritual abuse clients:** The nature of the trauma suffered by ritual abuse clients is extreme. You must be able to hear and help the client process physical, sexual, emotional, and spiritual abuse. Some of what you will hear will be bizarre and horrendous. You, as a professional, will have to be able to hear what is being said without overreacting or overpersonalizing it.

3. **Receive quality supervision on a regular basis:** I am a firm believer in professional group and individual supervision. This allows you to process your own reactions to the horrors about which you are told. Supervision also helps you to identify early the transference and countertransference issues that will inevitably occur. Never be afraid to ask for help. Teamwork is often the key to real success.

4. **Do not rush the processing of memories:** Have clients develop crisis plans, self-care techniques, support structures, and identify personal triggers before you begin the work of processing memories. Encouraging clients to remember their ritual abuse without laying a strong foundation is disastrous, not only for your client, but for you as well. Professional safety and client safety are issues you must develop before you begin.

5. **Hypnosis is likely to retraumatize clients:** Because of the similarity between hypnosis and the programming or brainwashing that most clients experienced as part of their abuse, hypnosis is more traumatic than it is helpful. Many people think that hypnosis will speed up the recovery process, when, in fact, I find it slows the process down, and in most cases encourages crises. There are a lot of other resources available to assist you in the healing process. I suggest symbolic media therapy like collage, art therapy, journaling, photo therapy, music therapy, movement therapy, and even some psychodrama techniques.

6. **Evaluate for and deal with life-threatening issues first:** Ritual abuse clients often come with a laundry list of other issues; some may be life-threatening. Issues such as eating disorders, self-mutilation, suicidal ideation, alcoholism, and drug addiction must be treated and under control before work on any ritual abuse issues or memory processing can begin.

7. **Remember how your client survived her/his ritual abuse:** Most clients survived their abuse by keeping the torture and pain a secret. That need to keep the secret is what allowed them to survive all these years and probably keeps them functioning to this day. Entering into therapy is going to challenge that basic survival skill. Don't ask for all the secrets to be disclosed until the client has developed sufficient coping skills to keep her/him going through these hard times.

8. **Realize your mistakes:** No one is perfect, and ritual abuse survivors really need to know this. Teach your clients that failure is part of the recovery process, just as much as memory processing, joy, sadness, and pain. As a therapist, remember your mistakes, so that you know what does and does not work.

9. **Recognize the power of suggestion:** Because of the programming and brainwashing experienced by survivors, many are highly suggestible. Do not encourage clients to read material on the subject of ritual abuse until they fully understand their own experience. Also, do not bring material you are studying or reading into a therapy session, because I believe that it tends to taint or discount the client's specific experience.

10. **Empower your client:** As I said earlier, your client *survived* the trauma. Recognize that! Do not foster a hyperdependence that will retard or prevent recovery. Recognize your client's personal power; hold it forth for them, and they will be stronger for it.

11. **Deal with the spiritual aspects of recovery:** Regardless of the client's spiritual orientation, spiritual issues *must* be addressed as part of recovery from ritualized abuse. Because rituals are almost always performed as a "spiritual ceremony," you must realize that the spiritual aspect of your client has been severely wounded. Spiritual issues cannot be fully addressed until the client has made significant progress in her/his recovery.

VOICES OF RITUAL ABUSE SURVIVORS:
Insights And Perceptions

Silent screams can now be heard. Finding words to communicate who you are and what happened to you can be compared to using a muscle that has been immobilized for a long time. It needs to be worked gradually and gently at first before getting back to normal use. These stories of surviving ritualistic abuse provide examples of how some people coped and held on when life seemed unbearable.

As you become aware of the reality of your family life, you may find the rules and teachings you have lived by for many years confusing or incomprehensible. Over time, you have probably invested a great deal of emotional energy in maintaining the rules that you created to help you forget the impact of your abuse. You must unlearn the dysfunctional thought patterns and replace them with survival skills that are healthy. This is very confusing because, while some of the rules are not completely wrong, they are obviously not helping you become who you want to be.

Whether you were ritually abused or not, you probably found ways to insulate and protect yourself emotionally and physically from the trauma. In childhood this constant need for self-protection often causes the victim to suppress emotions and become numb (or create alternate feelings and coping skills). These survival techniques almost always carry over into adulthood.

At this point, allow yourself also to examine what you did to survive during the abuse and what you are doing to survive now. Honor the skills that helped you to survive. It is all right to use the survival resources you've developed, as long as they are not self-destructive or life-threatening. Do not judge yourself; your survival skills served a valuable purpose at one time.

As you grow, you will find that you no longer have a need for certain coping methods. Unhealthy coping skills can only be replaced when you have found healthy replacements and when you can thank yourself for surviving. Have compassion for yourself—this journey does not last forever!

Wendy Ann Wood

SUGGESTED READING FOR RITUAL ABUSE SURVIVORS

These books are not meant to be a replacement for therapy. I encourage each of you to discuss reading this material with your therapist before you begin. I do not recommend reading ritual abuse material until you have processed your own memories. Whenever you are reading material on any subject, be aware of how you are feeling while reading. Stop reading any time you begin to feel uncomfortable or are experiencing triggers or flashbacks.

Breaking the Circle of Satanic Ritual Abuse:
Recognizing and Recovering from the Hidden Trauma
Ryder, Daniel. Minneapolis: CompCare Publishers, 1992. Written by a ritual abuse survivor and therapist, this book provides clear information on ritual abuse recovery but is strong reading. Proceed with caution.

Don't Make Me Go Back, Mommy:
A Child's Book About Satanic Ritual Abuse
Sanford, Doris; Evans, Graci. Portland, Oregon: Multnomah Press, 1990. This is a children's book that discusses one child's experience with ritual abuse in a day care setting.

Painted Black
Raschke, Carl A. New York: Harper and Row, 1990. This book includes a history of Satanic ritual abuse.

Combating Cult Mind Control
Hassan, Steve. New York: Park Street Books, 1988. This book covers categories of ritual abuse not related to Satanic cults and is strongly recommended.

Suffer the Child
Spencer, Judith. New York: Pocket Books, 1989. One of the first quality books to address the issue of ritual abuse of children.

Signs and Symptoms of Ritualistic Child Abuse
Gould, Catherine. Los Angeles: Los Angeles County Commission for Women, 1988. Gould is one of the founders of *Believe the Children* and an excellent resource for identifying ritual abuse in children.

Like Lambs to the Slaughter
Michaelson, Johanna. Eugene, Oregon: Harvest House, 1989. A Christian book that discusses ritual abuse issues clearly.

Be sure to check out additional resources in the *Partners in Healing* chapter and *Reading Guide* at the end of this book.

RECOMMENDED READING
FOR PROFESSIONALS

Ritual Abuse
The Ritual Abuse Task Force. Los Angeles: Los Angeles County Commission for Women, 1989. A booklet covering research on ritual abuse crimes. I recommend it with caution. For more information write to: 383 Hall of Administration, 500 W. Temple St., Los Angeles, CA 90012.

Mind Abuse by Cults and Others
Greek, Adrian; Greek, Ann. Portland, Oregon: Positive Action Center, 1985. Pioneers in ritual abuse recovery, the Greeks write about their personal and professional experiences. To purchase the book send $10.00 to: The Positive Action Center, P.O. Box 20997, Portland, OR 97220.

Children for the Devil: *Ritual Abuse and Satanic Crime*
Tate, Tim. New York: Metheun, 1991. Tate takes an investigator's approach to the subject and provides a substantial amount of information on childhood ritual abuse.

CHAPTER FIVE

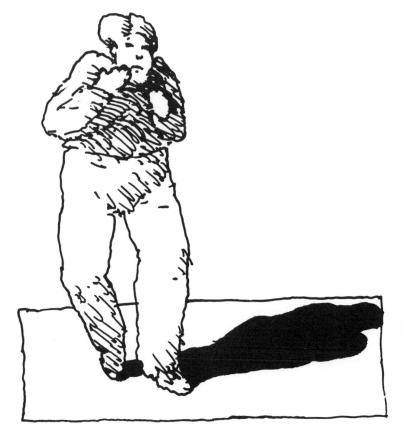

VOICES OF
MALE SURVIVORS

STATISTICS ON MALE SURVIVORS OF SEXUAL ABUSE

The majority of sexual abuse statistics previously discussed in this book include the abuse of boys. Following are some additional statistics that apply specifically to male survivors.

- One in seven males has been sexually assaulted by age nineteen (FBI, Uniform Crime Reports).

- 19 percent of perpetrators on males are female (Finkelhor, unpublished, 1986).

- More heterosexual than homosexual men are abusers (Mann, lecture notes, 1988).

- Male victimization involves more male-to-male sexual contact than female-to-male (Mann, 1988).

- Sexual desire has little to do with the motivation of male offenders when perpetrating sexual abuse on male children (Groth, 1982).

CHILDREN LISTENING

The wall too thin to muffle sounds
does not exempt the unintended listeners
the screech of bitter accusations,
lying, cruelty, infidelity, abuse.

Children cowering in disbelief.
How can they, those they love the most,
expose such hatred, threaten harm,
wear masks of fury, frightening?

Abandoned to bewilderment
thrust from the nest too soon
the world becomes a desolation.

No shields against the blasts of rage
no guides to seek a surrogate
no reason to believe
that anyone is otherwise.

D. Green

SMILEY

His schoolmates called him Smiley
though the involuntary grimace they saw
was more of pain than pleasure;
his eyes more like the fright of fear
than joy of anything.

Stunted he seemed a shrunken version
of an old disabled man
held to his desk by civil rules
though his unspoken wish was to crawl
away from ridicule or even kindness.

Later, those who read bestowed
a semi-literary title 'Scaramouche';
the repulsive grin took on texture
of botched surgery like keloid scars
teeth too aggressively exposed.

His teachers were impatient
annoyed that he was able unaided
to achieve as well as others.
They showed no sympathy why waste
a tear on a sufferer who smiles.

D. Green

INTERVIEW

Safe now the child rescued
from his loveless home
waits guarded to learn
about the "worker" whose task
is to repair his injuries.

He sits eye-contact avoided
shielding from intrusion
constrained response less said
less revealed too much so far
of pain that comes from telling
Trust a losing gamble.

There was no corporal punishment
No touching at all
his diet cold neglect his prison
cell a box of shrivelled silence.

In time some confidence restored
a few sad smiles withdrawal
less pronounced but both understood
the deepest scars never healed.

D. Green

WHO ARE YOU?

I had lost my innocence
Yet I am innocent.
He took my childhood
Away from me.

Made me his wife
Instead of his child.
Made me his chopping block
Instead of his bundle of joy.

Told me if I told
I would lose him — and Mom.
Told me if I told
I would be taken away
To a sad, ugly place
Called "Nowhere To Go."

So I became his wife.
Lost my innocence.
Carried his secret.
Gained his hatred.

And now I'm left knowing
Not knowing
The man I call
"Dad."

K. Kantola

WHAT'S THE MESSAGE?

father, you raped me
when i was a little boy
oh, so many times
then denied it many
times more.

now you leave me newspaper
clippings that say my former
gradeschool principal
(a 30-year-man like yourself)
raped many little boys
oh so many times over the years
and he and his family
deny it many times more.

and finally you leave me the one
clipping that says my principal
put a shotgun to his head
and expelled himself from life —
his family and friends still
maintaining his innocence . . .

what is the message for me
in those clippings? — a threat
not to tell or else you may do
the same? — or are you so
buried in denial you believe
i'm lucky i'm not one of his victims?
Are you aware that your other
son — my brother — is? . . .
What's the message?

K. Kantola

FROM DOWN THE HALL

outside my little hallway door
i hear the marital rape, "NO!
DON'T! GET OFF ME! Please . . ."
and then a helpless sigh
later
sobbing
    chocked down by coughing spells
        fading out halfway through the night.

months later she finds a
way to keep him off of her
so then he comes for me.
and i think, "good, at least
he's not doing this to her —
i'm saving Mom."

"take me, use me, abuse me —
just stay
away
from Mom!"

but what could she be thinking?
"thank god it's him and not me . . . ?"
or "there's nothing happening in
there — nothing."
who knows, who the hell knows —
Mom?

K. Kantola

A PROGRESS REPORT ON K. KANTOLA

It's been three and a half years since my first memories of abuse popped up. With the help of a therapist, support group, twelve-step group, and a couple of close friends I am now on the "other side" of the deep pain that had been running my life for the last twenty years. I am now out of therapy but in a twelve-step group as I continue working towards a full social recovery, and suspect I will be in this process for many years to come. Writing poetry for survivors' journals and small literary magazines has been an extremely important part of my recovery, as the printed word tends to validate my memories when I'm thinking "What if I just made this up." Also, the act of speaking out and being heard has empowered me, as now I feel my "speaking out" voice is louder than my perpetrator's "keep quiet" voice.

UNNAMED

I think about the years behind
And all the tears I've shed
The times of pain and agony
The days of slaying ten.

These memories and more do come
Each time I think of when
Within the night I scream in fright
His laughing from within.

M. Esham

NOT QUITE WHAT IT SEEMS

Sometimes his voice is still loud in
        my head
And I know that inside it will never
        be shed
But I've let go and let night slip away
So all he can do is speak until day

The things he wants and the dreams he
        bears
It all disappears, nothing more than
        nightmares
For when I wake up, beside me in bed
Is the mother Mary, my chest and her head

M. Esham

To My Flag I Bid Farewell

It was hard to be so insane
It was soul wearying to think of tortures
    for his body
My scars were broad pink strips
And my tears were made of blood let loose by
    an old razor
My mind became a playground of dreams and of
    a sad and deep melancholy
I missed the child who had never lived
The man who stood among you was a puppet
And the puppet master was an insane bastard
    using dreams as reality
I remember those days and think about my scars
For they are still there, strips of pink that
    shall forever mark me
But they will never again be my flag.

M. Esham

A PROGRESS REPORT ON M. ESHAM

I am back in school and am going to pass the eleventh grade.

SLEEPING BEAUTY

Laid out
Under a gauzy veil
Of sleep,
I feel the hall light strike
Me in the chest,
And I curl around it,
Roll away
Into dreams,
Away
From the creased frown
and darting, hungry eyes,
Hoping that this time,
The burning incandescence will fade
To cool, empty blackness.
But when the light dies,
It leaves a stirring in the dark
That cleaves to my dreams,
Breathes into them a rising, spinning life,
That smooths the wrinkles,
The eyes unchanged,
And I wish for a needle,
Immune to kisses,
To drain me for the last time
Of curse wakefulness
And heat.

Nelson G.

DIGGING IN THE GRAVE

I never missed you enough
to visit your grave,
yet here I am,
pounding, stake in hand,
sharpened,
through the serene web
the lush grass has laid
over the seeping earth.
Here,
trying to turn it,
realizing, finally,
the throbbing blood in my veins
is yours.

My feet have become horned,
gnarled and gripping,
so I need not feel
the harsh, dry dirt
humped at a distance
around the hole.

Mother still drops wilting
blue irises on your grave.
They, too, must turn to clear the debris
of so many years.

Approaching the pit,
on the edge of the glassy slope
wet with the still-hot blood;
I imagine the refuse gone,
and you spread your
arms
to me
in welcome.

Nelson G.

SURRENDER

Finally,
knowing the throbbing heat
in my veins
entered from the roots,

I release my grip
on the tree of my life,

Clothe myself
in the brightest robes
of my father's son,
and fall,
losing my colors in the rain,
passing my childhood
in those branches,
in the blight
I only now see beneath the rough bark.

And I drift
into the hole
the earth has opened for me,
resting at last
in the cool, fertile current
of the white stream
that rushes
under all.

Nelson G.

THERAPY

Taking the steps
down
I face
the blankness of smooth, sterile tiles,
polished,
slowly scarring,
bubbling
from the uneasy pools below,

And my fingers,
feel
the pools
dark
drops

As those fingers scrabble on the edges
to open

a vent,

for a scalding bath
to cleanse away
my father's son.

Nelson G.

A PROGRESS REPORT ON NELSON

I discovered just a year ago, in the process of therapy, that an adult molested me before I had seen very many years in this world. The process of being with that knowledge, and with the incest itself, has brought a great deal of pain and awareness into my life. My poetry has served both as a lens with which to see myself and as a tool of self-healing, although I believe the poetry originally dredged up the pain that brought me to therapy. I have, however, survived, and I am healing, and I feel grateful for that.

RECIPE FOR RECOVERY

Recipe requires one's own self.
1 cup of Hope
A dash of courage
2½ cups of trust
Several months of therapy
4 Tablespoons of faith
Work by the load
A bag of knowledge
A pinch of reassurance
A ton of support
One box of memories
2 pints of Higher Power
A handful of friends
1 platter of patience
Lots of time
A plate of mistakes
Stacks of affirmations
Buckets of tears
One Box of Crayons
A bunch of soft huggy things
1½ gallons of rewards
A good effort
2 big bags of understanding
Most important ingredient: LOVE

Constantly mix ingredients in your head. Let them rest in your heart at room temperature. Recipe will last a lifetime and can serve any amount to anyone.

R. Calderon

BARRIERS

I stand behind transparent walls,
barriers that keep me safe from them.
My memories are locked away in stalls,
so that they can never hurt me again.

I do not want to be exposed,
or be the brunt of cutting tongue.
I always have to seem composed,
the strength that always gets things done.

They cannot see me as I am,
for if they do, I'll soon fall prey,
my weakness like a wounded man,
will surely drain my life away.

This life I live but day to day,
my thoughts have no tomorrows.
Even my best days are shades of grey,
my laughter is sometimes borrowed.

Within my mind the demon roars,
clawing at stones I have erected.
In my fight I'm closing doors,
one each time I feel rejected.

But there is still this need of hope,
that this journey need not be bleak.
Perhaps today I'll begin to cope,
if I feel a kiss upon my cheek.

Raven

A PROGRESS REPORT ON RAVEN

I am a survivor of sexual and physical abuse. Sometimes it takes many years of hard work, honesty about one's self, and the deep desire to heal from within before the journey seems to pay a dividend. The ability to write about feelings, thoughts, and experiences has been therapy for me. This therapy has helped me to verbalize and share these thoughts with others who have had similar experiences. I hope that my poems will help others to open that door and to realize that healing, although sometimes painful, can be shared, and from sharing comes growth and strength.

VICTIM/OFFENDER

I have been a victim of sexual abuse, mental and emotional. I have also been the offender of sexual abuse, mental and emotional. I was with my physical mother for the first three years of my life. I know very little of those years except that she drank a lot and would end up leaving me in various places. These places were abandoned cars and alleys. The police would end up with me and she would take me back. Less is known of my physical father. I never met him.

During these first three years there was a great deal of emotional and physical abuse, the worst being that I did not learn the basics of love, caring, trust, giving and receiving. I also never learned the basic skills of being social. I experienced emotional pain, rejection, hurt and fear from those around me. I felt this to such a degree that I turned off my feelings and detached myself from them. Much had to be pushed inside.

Because of whatever abuse I was experiencing, my aunt and her husband adopted me at age three. These people raised me from this point until I was eleven years old, when my aunt died. I am sure now that if it was not for her care and love I would have become a much more destructive and dangerous sex offender.

During the years with this couple I showed many signs of needing serious professional help. I would laugh at times when my aunt would cry. Her sad feelings would reach me but would be twisted and not channeled in a healthy way. I would push people away, yet would not want them to go. I believe I began acting out my sex offender feelings at around five or six years of age. My adopted sister, who was much older than myself, would let me sleep with her from time to time. At one time, I tried to crawl up her nightgown — not being curious but in releasing some twisted feeling. She awoke and I got in trouble. I got some special attention.

Around age eight or nine, my acting out feelings went to those younger than myself. As I remember, this brought more special attention. I felt guilty and bad. At this same age, I, myself, was sexually abused by a much older male. Again I felt guilty for some reason, but I also felt good about the physical contact. It felt nice to be touched. From eight to fourteen years, I was abused by two more males. I lived in a world of guilt, feeling I was the only bad person around.

By the time I turned twelve, I had sexually abused three younger female children of families I was with. I also abused one younger male. When I was thirteen my stepmother, in an alcoholic condition, tried to seduce me.

My being emotionally and sexually abused as a child and adolescent was over. It was not until the age of twenty-three or twenty-four that I started sexually offending again, and this time the focus was on female adolescents and adults. This acting out started one year after I was married. I also started drinking alcohol again. I did not have any idea of my feelings inside or what was going on with me. I had no concept of my being a valuable person or that other people were valuable. I started acting out by picking up hitchhikers and ordering them to remove their clothes. I did this for a long time, then started exposing myself and other such forms of abuse. All this offending went on for one and one-half years. Then I was arrested for sexual abuse.

I was able to get into the only sex offender program in my state. Having the behavioral and emotional problems that make up most sex offenders, I also had the denial problems. I told myself and others that I would not offend again. I really believed this and meant it. Unfortunately, it was based on nothing. I had not made any changes or increased my knowledge of myself. Like any other serious problem, I didn't want to accept the part of me that hurt other people and myself.

I eventually was released and was back with my wife. Within a few months I was acting out again. I was returned to the hospital; I knew the games to play and was soon released. Within the year I was arrested again.

I was sent back to the hospital. At this point I had no idea what to do. Faking and lying my way through did not work, plus I did not want to hurt anyone else again. This time I did not move through the program for a number of years. During these years, with the help of many staff in the hospital, I slowly started making some very basic changes. Changes such as getting in touch with my feelings, accepting myself and being honest about what I'd done, handling feelings appropriately, and slowly learning to trust other people. This was very, very hard. It has all been hard.

Eventually I was released again. I have been out now for five years and have not harmed another person. I still have the ability to hurt others, but the changes I've made so far have kept my behavior constructive. I do many forms of volunteer work directed towards helping others help themselves. It is in no way easy but it is much better than what my life was before.

Merle

VOICES OF MALE SURVIVORS:
Insights And Perceptions

A tremendous burden is placed upon a child when she/he is in extreme pain and she/he has no one to support or help her/him. Boys in particular are forced to keep quiet about their abuse because they are socialized to believe that victimization and vulnerability is something that men should hide. Stereotypes of masculinity often force men to the seal away any indications of their abuse and bury them deep within themselves so that no one will see the lingering scars. You do not have to keep the secret any longer! Sexual abuse of males continues to go unreported; change can begin with you.

Keeping distressing secrets for a long time denies you the opportunity to be whole. It restricts your freedom to be you, because you are not sure who you really are. A part of you seems to be missing. This chapter shows the loneliness and isolation men experience as a result of being abused and societal pressures not to reveal that they were not strong enough to defend themselves — although they were only children.

Sometimes it is easier to cope with your experiences and feelings than to actually deal with the impact of your abuse. This may be because dealing is unfamiliar, while coping is what you learned at an early age. Understand that dealing happens gradually as you channel your energy toward taking care of yourself. Look at what you do to cope with the trauma and see if it is getting you what you really want and need. It is all right to keep the coping skills that are healthy and not destructive to yourself or others. Discard those habits that continue to hurt you.

It is important to begin to explore your abuse slowly, safely, and carefully. Let out some of these secrets in your own way and at a pace that is comfortable for you. This is a very scary thing to do, especially if you don't know what is there. As the feelings come, it may feel like you are losing ground, as you are overwhelmed by a flood of hidden emotions. Make sure that you have a support network. As you begin to trust them and yourself, you will be better able to deal with all that is locked away. Enter slowly into the darkness of the journey and carry your inner light with you. Know that you are not alone in this process.

Wendy Ann Wood

Suggested Resources For Male Survivors Of Childhood Sexual Abuse

Books

Victims No Longer:
Men Recovering From Incest and Other Sexual Child Abuse
Lew, Mike. New York: Nevraumont Publishing Co., 1988. This book was one of the first to address the issues of male survivors. Even though it is a few years old, it is really my first choice for male survivors.

Men in Pain:
Understanding the Male Survivor of Childhood Abuse
Cabe, Coe N. Aurora, Illinois: Aurora Counseling Clinic, 1989. A small paperback, packed with helpful information for male survivors and their supporters.

Adults Molested as Children:
A Survivor's Manual for Women and Men
Bear, Evan; Dimock, Peter T. Seattle: The Safer Society Press, 1989. A helpful manual written by and for survivors.

Men Surviving Incest
Thomas, T. San Luis Obispo, California: Launch Press, 1989. Written by a male survivor who incorporates his thoughts on the healing process with the slant of a twelve-step program.

Surviving with Serenity
Thomas, T. Deerfield Beach, Florida: Health Communications, Inc., 1990. Thomas, a survivor himself, writes in a thought-for-the-day style that is really wonderful.

Be sure to check out additional resources in the *Partners in Healing* chapter and *Reading Guide* at the end of this book.

Audio Tapes

Welcome To The World

Underwood, Judy K.: According to Underwood, "This tape will create the nurturing beginning your infant self deserves. You will experience profound acceptance as a male. *Welcome to the World* uses guided imagery to welcome your younger self to a new life filled with love and caring." We use this tape in our *Finding Your Inner Child* groups, and the participants have found it to be a very powerful tool. I recommend repeated use of the tape because we have found that new feelings emerge each time the tape is used. *Welcome to the World* allows survivors to work on getting in touch with their inner child, in a safe way, between therapy sessions. For more information contact: Odyssey, 1-800-733-6104.

CHAPTER SIX

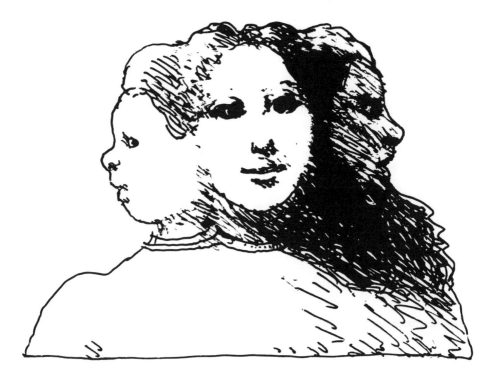

VOICES OF MULTIPLICITY

MYTHS AND FACTS ABOUT MULTIPLE PERSONALITIES

Myth: *People diagnosed with multiple personality disorder (MPD) are really schizophrenic.*
Fact: Schizophrenia and MPD are not the same diagnosis. While they are both characterized by auditory hallucinations (hearing voices that are not one's own), the voices multiples hear are their own internal alters. Schizophrenics, on the other hand, hear voices that are external. Schizophrenia is classified by the American Psychiatric Association as a psychosis, while MPD is considered a dissociative disorder.

Myth: *Multiples are really suffering from a form of mental retardation.*
Fact: Research has found multiples to be extremely intelligent; they are also considered to be extremely talented, organized, and creative. Being multiple is a creative form of self-protection from childhood sexual abuse.

Myth: *Most multiples are unable to function in society.*
Fact: Multiples maintain demanding jobs, care for families, and function in society. Remember that one of the main skills of multiples is to keep the MPD carefully disguised. The people they encounter in their daily lives see them as "normal" people.

Myth: *People with multiple personality disorder (MPD) are usually incurable.*
Fact: MPD is not an incurable disorder. With treatment, one of three different types of recovery is possible: 1) *fusion,* in which all of the alters or personalities are integrated into one personality; 2) *administration,* in which the core personality, or another strong personality, becomes the administrator of all the different personalities. Administration eliminates time loss because each alter accepts direction from the administrator. Skills are shared and there is open communication between the alters; 3) *partial integration,* in which the amnesiac boundaries of each personality are lifted and the alters make decisions about life cooperatively.

STATISTICS ON
MULTIPLE PERSONALITY DISORDER

- Sexual abuse, specifically incest, is the most frequently reported type of childhood trauma in patients with multiple personality disorder (MPD). This sexual abuse usually involves extreme forms of sadism.

- 10 percent of sexual abuse survivors and 2 percent of nonabused patients were found to carry the diagnosis of MPD (C.A. Ross, 1991).

- Most MPD patients report experiencing three or more different types of trauma during early childhood. This can include any combination of sexual abuse, physical abuse, ritualized abuse, and emotional abuse. P. M. Coons et al. (1988) found that 68 percent of the multiples in his study experienced sexual abuse; and 60 percent experienced physical abuse.

- 90.2 percent of multiples are female and 9.8 percent are male (C.A. Ross et al., 1990).

- 95.1 percent of multiples have had "extensive involvement with the mental health system" (C.A. Ross et al., 1990).

- There is some evidence which suggests that there is a period of time, from infancy to about age nine, during which children are most susceptible to developing MPD. This is thought to occur because children are more able to dissociate than adults.

- MPD patients are often repeatedly misdiagnosed. This is due, in part, to the fact that they present with other psychiatric symptoms in conjunction with the MPD. These symptoms include, but are not limited to insomnia, suicidal thoughts or actions, and depressive symptoms (Putnam et al., 1986); amnesia, fugue states, anxiety or panic attacks, and depersonalization (Bliss, 1984); substance abuse and auditory hallucinations (Coons, 1984). Patients frequently complain of physical symptoms for which there is no physical evidence (Waldschmidt, 1990).

- Diagnosing MPD is difficult and does not usually occur early in therapy. An average of six to six and a half years of therapy to arrive at a diagnosis is common in most literature (Putnam, 1989).

INSIGHTS ABOUT SURVIVORS WITH MULTIPLE PERSONALITIES:
What We Want You To Know About Us And Being Multiples

1. More often than not, we became multiple in response to an overwhelming trauma, which we either observed or experienced at an early age.

2. Becoming a multiple personality was a way to survive something awful. Please do not ask us to get rid of this coping skill until we have been able to replace it with something else.

3. Remember that multiplicity is woven into the fabric of terror. Our personalities split in order to avoid facing all of the fear at once. For integration to occur, we must confront the terror.

4. Multiple personality disorder is not a demonic possession. Please do not treat us as though there were something spiritually wrong with us.

5. Schizophrenia and MPD are not the same. We are not crazed or psychotic. We are creative, intelligent, and resourceful.

6. We used to believe that fusing, or integrating (that's putting all the people we are into one), would kill everyone off. That is not true! Parts that are fused do not go away or die, they just help us to get stronger. We rely on their skills to help us in our recovery, as we have done in the past; only now more of us know about them. After all, we are all really ME!

7. We do not like the word "disorder!" There is nothing disordered about what we did to survive. All the parts helped to keep us alive. We have to honor that before we can begin to heal. We are so thankful to each of our selves for doing the work to get us to today. Now we can become "I" and look forward to tomorrow.

8. Therapy for MPD does not take a few moments in time. We had to go through a lot of therapy just to be found. Now the real work begins. Please do not judge us while we go about the process of finding our selves.

9. Our childlike alters like to play. We invite our nonmultiple friends to join us, reassuring them that playing with us will not make them multiple.

10. We are not like Sybil or "The Enemy Within" so please do not treat us like that. We hold jobs, are parents, spouses, and friends.

THERAPY

I told
I listened
I forgot
I waited
I watched
I sought
I ached
I wept
I groaned
My questions
My chaos
I owned

He listened
He spoke
He knew
He waited
He watched
He was true
He reached
He opened
He cared
His hope
His trust
He shared

D. Johnson

GRIEVING

Finding sadness hidden well
Between lines of forgotten time
And stashed in seams of heart and mind.
I feel the gentle push, then a shuddering,
Rending in sudden birth I hear sorrow's cry
Helpless and dripping, I embrace and rock my soul.

D. Johnson

WEATHERED SISTER

I, your weathered sister, sail the winds of folly and fear.
    Woman/child astride a wooden horse racing across the hills,
    In scarlet gown, wispy, golden curls whipped about.
    Mother of lost caterpillars seeking protected
        Havens to weave their magic cocoons.
    Harlot of the village disdaining the mocking gaze from the
        church widows.
    Queen of sadness plundering the depths of
        Sorrow's lonely chasms.
I, your weathered sister, look across your kindly eye and
    Take down the sails.

D. Johnson

FRIEND

Uprooted and drying
Under the sun
For eyes to see.

Few would touch the mangled roots.

Only one
Gently placed the weathered tendrils
Back into the earth.

Only two hands held on
While the soil was watered
By choruses of weeping.

D. Johnson

SECRET PLACES

In deep caverns of her soul
Motions mysteriously grind
Quarreling, wrestling beneath her brow
Words she cannot find
Concentrating on things at hand
Upheaval and chaos rife,
Pulled and pressed she falls away
To the hands of a borrowed life.
Invisible, unknown yet seen,
Another lives another breathes
A passenger, a prisoner on a different trail
Silent she rides, alone she grieves.

Who is this child
What is this grief
I hear the whisper of her calling
From a place so far, so close;
Sometimes there is only silence
Sometimes there are only tears
Yet the presence running deeply
Reaches from the caverns through the cobwebs;
Warmth, the breath of life, the soft and silent strength
Buried way beneath the bitterness
Reaching out so tentatively
Hungry to learn the truth of love's security
Hoping only to heal and grow.

D. Johnson and Steve C.

A PROGRESS REPORT ON D. JOHNSON

I live in the Pacific Northwest with my husband, teenage daughter and younger son. During 1989 I was in and out of the hospital for five months, struggling with depression, anxiety and suicide. It was at that time I was diagnosed as having multiple personality disorder. I am in therapy and learning about ourselves and the impact abuse has had. I find writing and doing artwork very helpful in connecting things.

June's Acceptance

As time flies by and we live all alone
The memories of past no longer creep into the home
We now can live, my family and me
Seeking peace and acceptance of all there is to be.

There can be growth, there can be some healing
It may take years, but it all creates new feeling
Forgiving? No, but understanding, yes.
His part in all this he needs to confess.

I see sex abuse as a damaging part
Of lives of anyone who shares a confused heart
The memories are clear (for me) now as we believe
The times of fear and anger are soon to be relieved.

But not for everyone who hasn't come to this part
Of living and dying to memories with a strong start
Peaceful, attentive and solemn are days
But understanding his corruption he learned ways.

It could have happened to just K— that's me
But it probably happened to him as I now see.
He had to have learned all that he said and did
No way in the world could he do all this as a young kid.

But whether or not he learned it that way
I still won't know why it was done more than one day
I won't or can't forgive this brother of mine
He prolonged the agony of sex abuse for a long time.

K. Hopkins

A PROGRESS REPORT ON K. HOPKINS

Things are going slow in my recovery phase right now. I have been diagnosed as a multiple personality by an expert. I am leaving the life of one to be a part of many. I am now dealing with the memories of many and hope to return soon to "one." Thank you for letting us all share our pain. I thank you all for sharing your pain and recovery with us too. We are living each day with fear and strength and coming to believe little by little that it was not us that was to blame. We write poems, we cry, we hold onto each clear moment within our minds and realize it is then that the true K. Hopkins can come out safely without fear.

Things in my life are once again very difficult to endure — but I am doing it! As we learn about each other there is growth. My writings come from us all it seems — bits and pieces of my memory shared by the people inside my brain. Sometimes they remember more than I do and in ways protect me from any further harm. This is good. As I continue therapy I grow and accept who we all are and how we all relate to each other. This is all we can do.

I am happier than it ever seemed possible! I am in therapy dealing with the abuse that happened to me as a child. My therapist is a really great help to me. For the first time in the thirty-two years that I have been alive peace has finally found me. It is a good feeling to be sure of myself and others. This opportunity to write poems has given me the validation that it is okay to open up and talk about the abuse, and that is what I am most thankful for. I am okay and getting stronger by the week.

TREE

THE tree stands
silent and alone
gray, barren, lifeless

WRAPPED in silence
branches reaching to the unknown
tossed about by the winds of fear
doubting the existence of one who cares

SILENTLY he appears
touching the branches
with love and care

THE tree stands
suddenly not alone
branches reaching toward
the one who cares

GROWTH made possible
a single leaf
a sign of life

THE tree stands
wanting to be known.

Mary L.

SOME THOUGHTS FOR PROFESSIONALS WORKING WITH MPD CLIENTS

1. **Prepare for post-traumatic stress symptoms:** Most of the time, multiple personality disorder (MPD) clients do not have post-traumatic stress disorder (PTSD) symptoms until the trauma begins to emerge and is accessible to most, or all, alters. This usually does not occur until you are close to beginning the fusing process. Preparing clients for flooding and flashbacks before they occur is extremely helpful.

2. **Handle MPD clients in a nonthreatening way:** Clients with MPD have high startle responses so it is important that you do not do anything that may appear threatening. A raised voice or quick movement is likely to cause rapid personality shifts.

3. **Educate your client as to what the recovery process looks like:** For traumatized clients, it is often difficult to imagine what recovery looks like. Keep a road map for yourself and your client to assess those issues which have been processed and those which still need to be explored.

4. **Teach parenting skills:** Most clients with MPD do not have a good working knowledge of parenting skills. Some therapists find that teaching these skills as a part of therapy can assist the client in dealing with her own biological children and/or her child alters. There are also some quality books on the subject (see suggested reading for multiples).

5. **Address ways to maintain families during treatment:** For clients who have children, encourage them to seek occasional respite care. As with all partners of survivors, spouses of MPD clients need education to teach them how to help their partner in times of stress. I strongly recommend support groups for partners, where they can get support and work on their own issues.

6. **Assist clients in coordination of care:** Often clients are seeing their therapist, a psychiatrist for medication management, a physician, and other medical/mental health professionals. Due to the switching of alters, it is useful, and sometimes necessary, for the primary therapist to network among the professionals.

7. **Know the difference between severe disassociation and MPD:** Some therapists consider MPD to be synonymous with dissociation. It is my belief that dissociation is one continuum and multiple personality disorder is something altogether different. Clients with severe dissociation are seeking explanations to their behaviors and time loss — don't let MPD be the easy explanation. For someone who does not have the disorder, an MPD diagnosis can destroy their life, because it does not get to the core issues.

8. **Practice good self-care:** Never go to work emotionally hungry. Take care of yourself, seek regular supervision, have strong personal and professional boundaries, and finally, do not be so intrigued by your challenge to find the correct diagnosis that you loose sight of your goal: healing the survivor. Once you lose sight of this, the therapy is for your benefit and not for the client's.

VOICES OF MULTIPLICITY:
Insights And Perceptions

Multiplicity, while difficult to deal with, is a creative way of coping with a horrific past. Once alters begin to communicate among themselves and with the core personality, shock — and ultimately a sense of betrayal — is felt when you realize what happened to you. Especially difficult is the knowledge that the abuse should never have happened at all. You are likely to come face to face with a lie that has tricked you into believing that the abuse you suffered was okay, but remember that no matter how much you want to minimize or rationalize, abuse should never happen to anyone. No abuse is okay.

With the realization of this betrayal comes a deep sense of loss and confusion. Fantasies of your "wonderful family" and "wonderful life" can no longer be preserved. You begin to doubt yourself when your insides tell you something does not feel right and reality does not match up. Not only do you feel betrayed by your molester, you feel betrayed by your inner selves, who are telling you that what happened is your fault. Remember, no one is ever responsible, in any way, for the abuse they suffered.

This chapter may bring up a lot of unanswered questions about your own reality, about what was and was not okay. Perhaps it is time to challenge what happened to you and how life was meant to be. Talking about this with someone you trust, so that you can be grounded in that truth, may be invaluable for you now. It is cleansing to be angry. It is healthy to mourn the loss of what should have been. Allow alters the opportunity to express feelings that may have been reserved for only a few selves in the past. Proceed with love and gentleness.

Wendy Ann Wood

SUGGESTED READING
FOR MULTIPLES

These books are not meant to be a replacement for therapy. I encourage each of you to discuss reading this material with your therapist before you begin. Because many survivors with multiple personalities were ritually abused, I do not recommend reading ritual abuse material until you have processed your own memories. Whenever you are reading material on any subject, be aware of how you are feeling while reading. Stop reading any time you begin to feel uncomfortable or are experiencing triggers or flashbacks.

Can I Look Now? *Recovery From Multiple Personality Disorder* Downing, Rachel. Baltimore: Recovery Communications, 1992. This handwritten and illustrated pamphlet is by a female therapist who is recovering from multiple personality disorder. Her story is both simple and powerful in its portrayal of the recovery process. Downing provides hope, not only for those who have been diagnosed with MPD, but for all of us who at times feel "split off" from our feelings and ourselves. For additional information contact: Educational Recovery Communications, 1498M Reistertown Rd., Box 333, Baltimore, MD 21208, (410) 486-0141.

Multiple Personality Gift:
A Gift For You and Your Inside Family
Pia, Jacklyn M. Saratoga, California: R & E Publishers, 1991. This easy-to-read volume includes work for both child and adult alters. I recommend it for those who have been clearly diagnosed with MPD. Especially helpful is the chapter "Steps to Household Management." Distribution is limited. If it is not available in your area, contact the publisher at: (408) 866-6303.

Be sure to check out additional resources in the *Partners in Healing* chapter and *Reading Guide* at the end of this book.

RECOMMENDED READING
FOR PROFESSIONALS

Diagnosis and Treatment of Multiple Personality Disorder
Putnam, Frank. New York: The Guilford Press, 1989. An excellent
resource for therapists beginning to explore the issues of MPD clients. Putnam includes examples for laying the foundation for
working with clients.

CHAPTER SEVEN

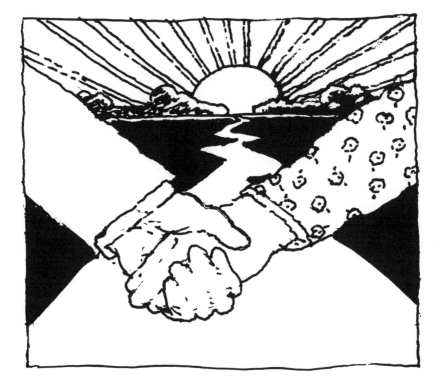

PARTNERS
IN HEALING

To Our Supporting And Intimate Recovery Partners:
What We Want You To Know About Our Sexual Abuse Recovery Process

Following is a collection of ideas written by survivors for support people in their lives. Remember that not everything listed applies to every survivor. You might want to discuss the list with the person you are supporting. See which items apply to them and their recovery process, and identify those which you, as a supporting partner, will be able to follow through on.

FOR SUPPORTING
RECOVERY PARTNERS

1. Please do not push me for more information than I can comfortably give you at any one time.

2. Let me go at my own pace. I know the best speed for my recovery process. Please honor that.

3. I need a lot of understanding and support from you, although it may not always be fair to expect it.

4. If something happens to trigger memories or flashbacks, I need to be accommodated, although I may not always know what I need because I don't have a lot of control over my emotions.

5. I don't want to feel shame or judgment from others. Please believe me when I tell you things. Please accept me. If you do not believe me, at least tell me so — it is a lot easier than having someone lie to me.

6. Please realize that recovery is long and involved and requires a lot of hard work. There are no "quick fixes" and no magic wands.

7. It helps me if you realize that memories are deep, painful, and slow to be processed.

8. Please don't say to me, "It couldn't have really been all that bad." It was! Discounting or minimizing my abuse experience fosters my own denial and hinders my recovery.

9. Know that it takes a lot of energy to do this work.

10. Learn the warning signs of self-abuse, and when you see them in me, remind me of the coping methods I can use to keep myself safe.

11. Realize that you can not "fix it," but you can be there for me.

12. Encourage me to seek professional help as needed, because sometimes I lose sight of reality.

13. When I am flooded with memories of abuse, I appreciate having someone available who can help protect me from my terrifying thoughts and emotions. However, I usually can't accept being touched. If my impulse control and judgment are impaired, I may need you to help me stay safe.

14. Please tell me if you feel unable or unwilling to give me support when I ask for it. Saying you are there for me when you are not is a recapitulation of my abuse.

FOR INTIMATE RECOVERY PARTNERS

1. My sexual abuse has greatly affected my ability to trust my intimate partner.

2. I often feel unlovable and unworthy of your care and support.

3. I need you to be motivated to work on your *own* issues, to grow and change individually, as well as on our "couple" issues.

4. I have trouble integrating emotional and physical intimacy. My history of abuse makes these experiences mutually exclusive.

5. I want you to be involved in a therapy group (professional or self-help) that will teach you about being the partner of a sexual abuse survivor. I do not have the energy to do my own recovery work and teach you at the same time. You also need your own support system that you can turn to in your own time of need.

6. While in the early stages of sexual abuse healing, my interest in our sexual relationship is likely to change. Please be patient. If you want to discuss your concerns about our sexual relationship, please ask me, but respect my decision not to talk about it at that moment.

7. Please ask permission for hugs and kisses. Unexpected affection can put me into a flashback or body memory.

8. Your willingness to read material about my recovery process is a sign that you care about me.

9. There are times when therapy may have been so difficult or painful that I may not want, or be able, to talk about it.

10. Abandonment is my greatest fear when it comes to our relationship. Please tell me, only if you truly mean it, that you will be with me through this painful time in my life.

11. I need to be reassured of the feelings you have for me.

12. I need you to be willing to discuss and negotiate around sexual needs.

13. Please understand that I often have limited energy and time during some of the stages of my recovery process.

14. There are times when I need more physical space than other people. Often when I say, "Don't touch me!" I am not really talking to you. Do not take it personally, but please honor my request.

Effects Of Sexual Abuse On An Intimate And/Or Committed Relationship

Below is a list of some of the effects incest and sexual abuse can have on a committed relationship. Obviously, the effects are not the same for every couple, and they depend upon a variety of factors including duration and frequency of the abuse, severity and type of abuse, age at which abuse began, the relationship between the offender and the survivor, and the response of others if the survivor reported the abuse.

When using this list, identify those which apply to you and realize that you are not alone in your struggle.

- Difficulty with intimacy
- Lack of satisfying sexual relations
- Periods of unexplained rage
- Emotional detachment
- Hypersensitivity to touch
- Flashbacks or "spacing" during sex
- Avoidance of sexual feelings
- Withdrawal from social and sexual interaction
- Sabotage of healthy relationships
- Indiscriminate choice of partners
- Low sexual desire
- Inability to trust the partner/relationship
- Inability to allow closeness
- Feeling trapped in the relationship
- Painful intercourse
- Sporadic sexual satisfaction
- Sexual misinformation
- Lack of good, clear communication

- Feeling obligated to engage in sex
- Lack of emotional bonding
- Feelings of sexual exploitation
- Guilt feelings about sex
- Avoidance of addressing sexual concerns
- Hypervigilance and alertness
- Overreaction to "minor" life events
- Irrational guilt
- Feelings of isolation and neediness
- Denial, avoidance, repression
- Low stress/anxiety tolerance
- Feeling helpless and hopeless
- Nightmares and insomnia
- Viewing sex as "bad" or "evil"
- Childlike interactions
- Self-hatred
- Limited knowledge of sexual or personal boundaries
- Projecting feelings of hostility, etc., toward the offender onto the partner
- Inability to distinguish loving, nurturing sex from exploitative sex
- Enjoying sexual contact only after penetration has occurred
- Avoidance of sexual acts experienced during abuse

BILL OF RIGHTS FOR PARTNERS OF SURVIVORS

1. The right to a definition of what you see as the rules for our relationship
2. The right not to be defined as an abuser
3. The right to my own feelings and the need to express them
4. The right to take care of myself
5. The right to fail occasionally as a supporter in your recovery
6. The right to trust and be trusted
7. The right to be angry
8. The right to take some time out
9. The right to care about you
10. The right to see myself as an indirect victim of the abuse you suffered
11. The right to share in the healing process
12. The right to be angry at the offender(s)
13. The right to be confused by new boundaries in our relationship
14. The right to explore and set my own personal boundaries
15. The right for us, as a couple, to experience peace in our lives

CAN'T SAY

I can't say I LOVE YOU
for fear you'll run away
I can't say my feelings
for it is me they will betray.
I can't say I want you forever more,
for fear you will close that BIG DAMN DOOR.
I can't say my heart is breaking . . .
trying to hold these feelings inside.
I know you would admit how very hard I've tried.
I can't forgive the bastard,
who has done these things to you . . .
But most of all I hate the fact,
He can ruin love so true.

Brave Star

INCEST SURVIVOR CHOPPING ONIONS

White onion on the wooden cutting board,
its taste on your fingertips —

Metal slicing skin to wood
metal slicing skin to wood —

Years of trees, the sun falls away
under a swing set

How many sour secrets?
How many pairs of loving eyes?

The kitchen clock strikes seven,
your cheeks streaked with tears

Metal slicing skin to wood—
too many meals have been like this

Outside, a brown-eyed girl
scatters the leaves with a playful kick

R. Lovitt

SOMETIMES THE KNIGHT
(This Poem Is For Those Who Go Through Our Pain With Us)

Sometimes the knight
grows weary
With fending off the night
and the terror of it.
Grows tired of
the inexhaustible distress
of damsels who are needy
without wanting, who are passionate without desire
whose stark eyes tell more
than one wants to hear,
whose prisons are themselves
whose dragons are elusive
and never finally slain.
Sometimes the knight
must defend his own honor
against those who find him
and name him champion
and then
can't believe him.
Sometimes the knight
cries "Enough!"
at the bottomless need
of his dark ladies;
at their spiraling descent
at their retreats at night.

And in the afternoon
instead of being
for God's sake just there,
and okay for once,
Sometimes the knight
doubts his calling
when the damsel's desire to die
so real and so imagined
Invades him.
He knows how few bandages he's got
and that he must prop
the frail crutch
of belief in the knight
up under the chasm
that seeks not to know herself.
Sometimes the knight
must rescue himself
and rest from the quest of the grail.
He feeds himself steak and stiff bourbon,
watching the game
he waits
for the next call to rescue.

Sandra Joel A.

FACING FEAR

Fear seen in serious eyes
Fear felt in timid heart
Fear denied preferring dying
To the pain of futile trying
Yet there lingers hope and courage
Lost love, a sweet delusion —
Or could there be a string of something
Far beyond the rotten roots
Deep decayed, artifacts of history
Fragile structure, illusions starting
to be seen.

Fear feeds upon some distance
On lonely time, resistance,
On shameful scars of pain
Or rumination of rejection
Trust betrayed, humiliation
Of innocence remembered
Lost, but not to blame.

Acceptance offered
Love received
Tentative
The risks so sensitive
The hurt so deep
"Tread lightly on this fragile someone"
So protection said so softly
"Let me keep my secrets for a while"
Yet time's demands
The power to provide
Would ride the winds of fortune
Risking further fear
Upon this painful path
You need not go alone.

Steve C.

At The Cusp

Fear gripped as
The thoughts of loss
Settled into time
Time filled with empty questions
Scenes of common horror
Of simple choices gone awry.

Hope prevailed
As cusp is come to
Power realized
In a way thus unexpected
Simple in its purity
Just a taste
Of more to be.

Steve C.

A PROGRESS REPORT ON STEVE

I am a psychologist in Pendleton, Oregon, and past president of the Oregon Psychological Association. Writing has been a hobby for years. It is wonderful to be published when one has something to say. The hard work done by my clients and others is an inspiration which asks me to express these thoughts and feelings.

PARTNERS IN HEALING:
Insights And Perceptions

It is hard to accept that someone you care about so deeply has been sexually abused! It is natural to feel the deep sense of loss, and sadness that accompanies this realization. Feel the anger, the loss, and the myriad of other emotions. Realize that there is nothing you can do to change what has gone before. Your impact begins now. Deal with your own issues about sexual abuse, care giving, intimacy, and others that will emerge during this time.

Remember, it is likely that the survivor you support did not have their basic needs met, needs like love, nurturing, and an honoring of the developing self. You cannot recapture what they did not get, no matter how hard you try. Survivors can never go back and be that child again, but with this realization also comes an opportunity to help the survivor find the nurturing parent inside her/himself. Modeling is often the best way to teach this skill.

Remember that sexual abuse is very confusing, because in our adult world sexual intimacy is symbolic of true love. A child who is forced, either overtly or covertly, to participate in abuse is receiving mixed messages. How can something that is supposed to represent love be so traumatic and painful? As supporting partner, or intimate partner, you must rely on others to provide you emotional comfort, and frequently you must look inside to get your needs met. You must be your own best friend. Care for yourself. Listen to yourself. Accept yourself. Once you have done this, you will be ready to hear the story of your partner's abuse and take part in her/his recovery.

We are on this earth together. Strength comes from relying on and helping others. Having a partners' support group or therapist to support, guide, and teach you is very helpful. Remember, there are good times in recovery and there are difficult times; if you are willing to make a commitment to be a support person in a survivor's life, you must be there for both.

Wendy Ann Wood

SUGGESTED RESOURCES
FOR PARTNERS AND SURVIVORS

Survivors of abuse often find it extremely difficult to talk about a variety of issues related to intimate relationships. The following is a list of books and tapes which can be helpful in facilitating communication. While there are others out there, I believe that these are the best. I strongly encourage partners and survivors to read the material together and talk about the issues raised.

Books

The Sexual Healing Journey
Maltz, Wendy. New York: HarperCollins, 1991. An excellent book for survivors, which includes information for healing with an intimate partner.

Incest and Sexuality: *A Guide to Understanding and Healing*
Maltz, Wendy; Holman, Beverly. New York: Lexington Books, 1987. This was the first book to openly discuss incest and issues of sexuality. I use the "Dating and Sexual Behaviors" list in groups, and participants find it helpful in the process of clarifying their wants and wishes.

Survivors and Partners:
Helping the Relationships of Sexual Abuse Survivors
Hansen, Paul A. San Franciso: Heron Hill, 1991. An excellent book written for partners and survivors to further understanding of the effect childhood sexual abuse has on a relationship. The author, also a survivor, alludes to male survivors, but fails to use nonsexist language.

Ghosts in the Bedroom: *A Guide for Partners of Incest Survivors*
Graber, Ken. Deerfield Beach, Florida: Health Communications, 1991. This book addresses some issues for partners of multiples that seem to be lacking in current publications. I include this book with some hesitation because of Graber's over-generalizations,

which appear throughout the book. It does, however, contain some helpful insights. Be sure to bring up questions you may have about this, or any other book, with your therapist.

Struggle for Intimacy
Woititz, J.G. Deerfield Beach, Florida: Health Communications, 1985. While this may be an older book, not specifically directed to survivors of sexual abuse, I believe that the message is one that is important to everyone.

Be sure to check out additional resources in other chapters and in the *Reading Guide* at the end of this book.

Videotapes and Audio Tapes

Partners in Healing:
Couples Overcoming the Sexual Repercussions of Incest.
Produced by Wendy Maltz, Steve Christiansen, and Gerald Joffee. An excellent videotape showing three couples in various stages of their personal healing. Two female and one male survivor share their stories. The only drawback of this tape is that it makes recovery look like a "quick fix." For additional information contact: Independent Video Services, 401 E. 10th St., Eugene, OR 97401, (503) 345-3455. It is also available in major video rental stores.

The Isle Of Pleasure: *Your Path to Sexual Fulfillment*
Underwood, Judy K.; Gaynor, Pamela A. This series of six audio tapes is for the female survivor who is beginning to explore her sexuality. The sixth tape involves listening to the tape with your partner. If you are ready to begin to get in touch with your body, from which you may have been detached for many years, this is must listening! The tapes are tastefully done, empowering, and give the listener the permission needed to explore her own sexuality. For more information, or to place an order, contact: Odyssey, 515 S. Sherwood St., Ft. Collins, CO 80525, or call 1-800-733-6104.

CHAPTER EIGHT

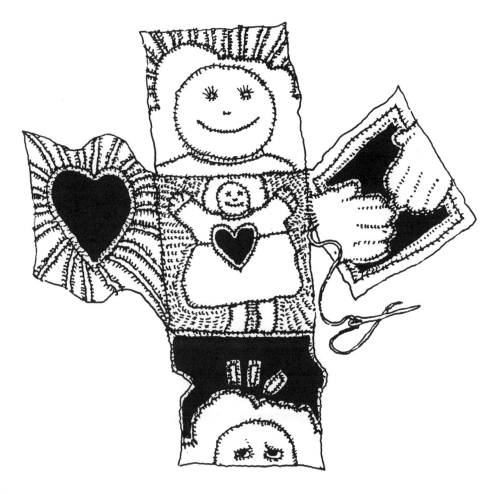

THE HEALING
PROCESS

JOURNALING:
A Tool To Journey Inward

In the beginning of the healing journey, most survivors are not aware of their feelings, except when they are extreme. Many sexual abuse survivors truly believe that they are going to die when they begin to feel for the very first time. The important thing to remember is that no one ever died because they had a feeling. Many people survived their sexual abuse by denying what was happening to them and by denying their feelings. Honor this denial because it was a survival skill. Journal writing helps survivors to express feelings, deal with denial, focus on the future when the moment seems dark, and communicate with significant others. No matter where you are in your recovery process, writing can provide a way to get in touch with the emotions of the day, or your thoughts and feelings about your own recovery. Following are some things to consider when journaling:

Why be in touch with feelings?

In order to tolerate the pain brought on by the trauma of childhood sexual abuse, you may have needed to suppress your negative feelings and concentrate entirely on survival. As adults many survivors use the same coping strategy to handle the problems of everyday life. But denying feelings and thoughts that occur in your life takes its toll on you, physically as well as emotionally. You must begin to get in touch with your personal pain in order to move from a victim to a survivor mentality, and then from surviving to thriving. I hesitate to rely on the old saying "no pain no gain," but it is really true.

Why keep a journal?

Journaling can be a barometer of your recovery journey. If you keep your journals, you will be able to look back on the progress you have made. Each time you write, you have the opportunity to know you, the writer, better. Journaling can help you to identify patterns in your recovery. You can see what worked for you and what didn't.

Writing gives you a chance to reflect on the positive things that you may be ignoring in life. Journaling can be used as a tool in the healing process, as it can be used to provide direction in the therapy setting and pinpoint changes you would like to see in your life. It is also a way for you to be aware of those around you who may be good people to add to your support structure.

For most survivors, the general level of trust in people, let alone their therapists, is low. I think it is important to bring your journal into therapy sessions. I often have a client who comes in and says, "I can't tell you this, but here, read it." I do not always make a point of reading client's personal journals during the therapy time. Usually, I ask clients to read a piece from their journal or share a summary of it with me, but that is all. Remember that the journal is yours and you are trusting your therapist with a very important aspect of your life.

People often ask me what to do with a journal once they have finished it. Some people throw them away, but I recommend keeping completed journals. If you worry about your journals being found, rent a safe deposit box in which to store them. Don't give your journals to your therapist for safe keeping. While she or he may be the only person in your life you can trust, I just don't think it's a good idea. It fosters a hyperdependence on the therapist. I have heard some clients say that leaving their journals with their therapist is like leaving a little bit of themselves there. Leave something else there, but not your journals. Again, I encourage you to be in charge of keeping your own journals secret if they need to be secret.

How does journaling assist in the recovery process?

I asked some of my clients this question, and they had great answers: "Journaling allows me to track issues to discuss in more detail with my therapist. I am better able to contain my emotions and behavior. Sometimes I can get a valuable measure of progress by reviewing things I have written over a period of weeks and months." This client uses her journals as a containment tool. Sometimes during flooding, survivors cannot break out of their thoughts and/or emotions. What happened then and what is happening now seem to all mix together.

Another client said, "Journaling enabled me to communicate with myself and my therapist much more effectively. By journaling my thoughts, I was less likely to forget what I needed to talk through with her. Those things had a nasty way of 'slipping my mind' on occasion." The mind has a built-in defense system: the denial mechanism. That "slipping my mind" syndrome is the mind trying to take care of you in times of distress, but it's not always helpful when you are trying to make progress in therapy.

A third client said, "I notice that when I have not been writing for a while, I feel bogged down, and journaling releases those feelings for me. Journaling has helped me to track my progress for the years and months that I have been going to therapy." Another client said that journaling "helped to get what I saw and felt out of my head and freed me up to let it go and not dwell on the material. Later, it was easier to share what was going on for me with my therapist or partner." Some people have intrusive thoughts that they cannot seem to get out of their mind. It's kind of like getting a song stuck in your head and never being able to sing anything else. The same goes for memories — by placing them in your journal you can tell yourself, "This is important material; I am writing it down so it is not forgotten, but I cannot deal with it now." This is an excellent self-care tool.

What about journaling for multiples?

Many sexual abuse survivors develop divided personalities in order to deal with past hurts and the new, unknown circumstances of today. The average nonmultiple survivor behaves differently with different people throughout the day, while a multiple will just switch personality states. Often multiples find themselves alternating between victim and survivor roles, the personal and professional roles, the typical parent, adult child roles of everyday life. Journal writing enables your divided self to note how many people you have been today and what all your thoughts, feelings, and options are in your present situation.

I encourage my clients to use a variety of colors for journal writing. The risk-taker alter might write in red, the conservative alter in black, the childlike alter in purple. As a result, both you and your therapist get a clear sense of how many people are on "your committee," who they are, and when they agree and disagree. As the chairperson of your personality, you can learn to make better choices, taking into account all aspects of who you are. When you are aware of the aspects of your personality, it is more likely that you will learn to make decisions you can live with.

How to keep a journal

A journal can be a place to list events of the day, but perhaps it is better to share flashbacks, feelings, concerns, opinions, and reflections on your personal recovery or on life in general. For those of you who don't know how to start, I suggest you begin by writing down events that elicited strong feelings. For those of you who do not even experience strong feelings, write down your goals, fantasies, and dreams.

Pick a special, comfortable, quiet place in which to write. It should be a place where you feel safe to express as much of yourself as you want. I like soft chairs, a candle, warm peppermint tea or a cold lemonade, and some mellow music. Make your writing place the same place every day if possible; that way it will become a safe haven for you in a sometimes stressful world.

You don't have to write everyday, although that probably is the most effective way for you to tune in to the fine details of your feelings. Survivors who are perfectionists may find journaling stressful. If you can get through the initial discomfort of not being rigidly structured, you will find it to be a great help. A client told me, "I told myself that I didn't have to write every day. I can write anywhere from one word to many pages, as I see fit. I gear it to my own unique method, because after all, it is for me and only me or those I choose to share it with."

I often find it is best to start clients out by writing every day for a month or two and then they can decide what pattern works best for them. Some people do more journaling in a single weekend at the beach than they did the entire three weeks prior. However, when I assign clients journaling homework, I expect them to do at least five days of work in the journal each week. Remember, journaling does not have to be all words and writings, it can be drawings and doodles too. It is also a place for play. Some clients find it a perfect space for small magazine collages. This is especially helpful for survivors who were abused when they were very young, and may not be able to verbalize or write about what happened to them.

One client said, "It is easier for me to journal when I keep reminding myself that I do not have to write every day. It is also helpful to remind myself that I don't have to write what would be pleasing for others. My journal is my life, and it includes everything from what my abusers did or said to my feelings about everyday things."

Everyone asks me, "What should I write in?" I encourage you to use something with bound edges like blank books, or bound drawing books rather than a binder/looseleaf type. Your journals need to be something special to you; if you do not feel special or welcome there, you are less likely to stick to it. So spend a little money, go down to the local stationery store, and find the kind of journal you want to write in. I like a book with fabric covers or the bound drawing books because of the thickness of the paper. I also favor those with lines on one page and blank paper on the opposing page, because they tend to be less restricting. Write with something you enjoy writing with, whether it is a fountain pen, a felt tip or a pencil. The "pilot varsity" is my favorite. It comes in several colors.

Whatever form journaling takes for you, it is often one of the most important tools in the therapeutic process. It allows you to journey inward to find out who you are and who you have the potential to be.

STAGES OF RECOVERY

Every person in a therapeutic relationship should be familiar with the stages of recovery. Use them as path markers — where you are going and what you have already covered — but please do not take this to be an immutable model of the recovery process. Recovery is different for every survivor. You know how best to heal yourself and you must honor your own recovery process. You know what is best for you and how fast or how slow you need to go. Trust yourself in this journey.

Recovery is not a process that happens in a linear fashion, each stage appearing in an orderly sequence. Instead, you may find yourself in stage three, moving on to stages four and five and then back to stage two again. That is not a failure, it is a part of the recovery process. You will find yourself working through several stages again and again, because when you are in any given stage, you work through the material you can safely process at that time. If there is more to work through, you will return to that stage until the trauma has been completely processed.

Stage One: Recognition of differences

You begin to notice ways in which your life is emotionally different from those around you. You begin to realize that not everyone feels the intensity of pain you are experiencing. You recognize, in some small way, that the sexual abuse you have experienced "may" have affected your life after all. You might see depression, control issues, sexual dysfunction, difficulty in maintaining healthy, positive relationships, an inability to deal with stress, workaholism, continually finding yourself in the role of victim, staying excessively busy in order to avoid dealing with feelings or thoughts that may occur, and unexplained rage. At first, you tell yourself that it is the result of something else, but in reality, your behavior is directly related to your abuse history. This is scary, but it is the first step to recovery!

Stage Two: Acknowledgment of issues

Now that you realize there is a problem, you seem unable to deal with what is going on in your life. Something specific may happen to make you come face to face with the fact that something is wrong. For most, acknowledgment occurs right before they seek therapy. In the past you may have considered your abuse to be "a little static," but now it has become "a sonic boom." This awakening may be caused by a major life event — a birth, death, marriage, losing a job or getting a promotion — or it may come when everything external in your life seems to be settling down: your children return to school, your job is secure, a crisis has passed. Unconsciously, you know that it is safe to work on your abuse issues now. Either way, acknowledgment is part of the process.

Stage Three: Searching for trust

Stage three involves the process of finding someone whom you believe you will be able to trust, while sharing all the thoughts and feelings you have kept stored away for many years. I am not speaking of a complete trust — that comes much later. I am talking about a inner knowing or gut response that tells you that it may be possible to trust this person, even if that trust is only the size of a speck. You may turn to a therapist or counselor, or someone else who has experience in sexual abuse recovery. That person should gather some general history and provide you with a basic education about sexual abuse recovery. You should know what to expect in the process you are about to begin. Learn the stages of recovery and discuss them in detail. This way you will not be caught off guard when something happens that you do not understand, like flooding or flashbacks. You should establish goals for therapy that relate to your specific needs and behaviors. Discuss long- and short-term support and treatment issues. Explore how secrecy was used as a weapon against you. Understand the concepts of personal and professional boundaries. Finally, your therapist should shine the light of hope on the road ahead. This is not an easy process. Remember, the first person you seek out may not be the right person for you. Keep looking until you find the person who fits your needs.

Stage Four: Telling your story

You will return to stage four many, many times. The true purpose of this stage is to recall each of your known abuse experiences verbally and connect them with the feelings you had to suppress while the abuse was happening. At first you might tell your story with little or no feeling, but do not worry. As you build trust with your therapist, you will become more aware of your feelings, and eventually you will be able to connect those feelings to your abuse experiences. Some people do not know how to go about sharing their story. I use the following guidelines with some of my clients. First, try to focus on just one offender and one abuse event. Then answer these questions: Who was your offender? How old were you when abuse by this person began? When did it end? How old were you when the event you are about to share occurred? Describe, to your own comfort level, what happened to you? Was anyone else there while you were abused? Did you ever tell anyone about this before now? If so, when, and how did that person respond to you? Do you still see your offender? If your offender was a member of your family, what is your relationship like with the rest of the family? What feelings do you have toward your offender? What feelings are you having right now, after sharing your story?

Telling your story helps to break the isolation and secrecy you have been carrying for so long. Work to your comfort level, then push yourself a little way into the discomfort, and then return to your comfort level. This will help you gain more control of the feelings when flooding begins.

Stage Five: Identifying coping skills

As you share your abuse history, it is likely that your old coping skills will come into play and try to protect you. In response to the vulnerability and fear you may feel while telling your story, you may experience denial, claiming that the abuse did not really happen, or that what did happen was really not all that bad; shame, a reflection of your own sense of innate badness, worthlessness, self-hate, and self-blame; guilt, in which you see a specific action or behavior and then evaluate it as wrong or bad; addictions, such as wanting to smoke, eat, drink, purge, or drug yourself into numbness;

physical illness, such as asthma, migraines, gastrointestinal and gynecological difficulties, and muscle tension; isolation, remaining alone with the truth of your abuse so that you convince yourself that you have no knowledge of it, and therefore, it never occurred; disassociation, which causes you to "space out," lose time, or for multiples, a different personality might emerge to take over your consciousness; self-mutilation, cutting or burning yourself as a way to externalize the internal pain; psychological symptoms, including depression, phobias, paranoia, suicidal thoughts, and panic attacks; and numbing, total or partial detachment from your body and emotions.

Once you have identified your coping skills, you have made a major step in your recovery. Remember, you cannot change old coping styles right away. Honor yourself for the way you survived the abuse and discuss with your therapist coping styles you want or need to replace.

Stage Six: Dealing with flooding

Flooding is what happens when the emotional impact of the abuse hits you full force. You begin to experience flashbacks that force you to face the denial of your abuse, if only for a few moments. You may have difficulty differentiating between the past, when the abuse was happening, and the present, in which you are an adult and, hopefully, safe from the abuses that you are remembering. Flooding can occur at any time and may take the form of visual memories, in which you actually see the abuse that happened; body memories, in which your body feels the aches and pains that are associated with abuse; auditory memories, caused by a certain smell, sight, sound or touch; and twilight dreams, those memories that occur just as you are falling to sleep or waking up. To cope with flooding you need to have close at hand your list of things you are going to do to take care of yourself while you are feeling so vulnerable. Review with your therapist the things you plan to do when flooding occurs. She/he will be able to help you choose safe and/or less toxic coping skills. Remember, doing something for someone else is not taking care of yourself. A flashback will always try to convince you that it has control over you and that you are powerless; but remember, it does not have to be that way. Develop skills to help you gain control over flashbacks.

Stage Seven: Development of self

Because childhood sexual abuse survivors are abused at such an early age, they spend their childhoods protecting themselves rather than developing their identity and self-esteem. Skills like separateness, nurturing, considering your own needs first, self-esteem, and self-worth were put aside while you concentrated on survival. To protect yourself, you may have created a false self to project to the world around you. Externally, this false self may look like over-achievement, perfectionism, competitiveness, rebelliousness, negative specialness, and/or the need to fail. Internally, the false self fosters denial, guilt, shame, lack of assertiveness, keeps the abuse a secret, maintains the view of the ideal family and ideal life, and a lack of self-esteem and self-worth except when helping someone else. Until now, this is all you have known, so you do not see it as a false self. After all, you have worked all your life to develop into who you are. When you realize that there is a false self, you begin to have a pervasive fear of having no identity. Be assured that there is a true self under all the false projections. During this stage you work at finding out who your true self is. In the same way a teenager does, you may experiment with different styles, attitudes, and behaviors. I have a client who says, "Oh no, not adolescence again!" every time she finds herself in this stage. But never fear, you will grow out of it.

Stage Eight: Feeling the grief

Grief is a pivotal point in the recovery process. In grieving, begin to realize that there are many things that were lost as a result of your abuse. This is a painful stage. Now is the time to examine your family. Grieve for the loss of the family you thought you had, but did not. Realize that your childhood viewpoint of the idealized family and ideal life was not a reality. Harder still is accepting the fact that your family, with whom you may still want a relationship, is not willing to cooperate in rebuilding the relationship. Other issues to explore may be personal loss including, but not limited to, parts of your emotional, sexual, spiritual, intellectual, intuitional, and physical selves (while it is possible to regain much during recovery, what *is* lost is the time you have spent without those aspects of your self), and the nature of the trauma. Recognize the full extent of the abuse and feel the impact it has on your life. This involves releasing the guilt and shame you have carried with you, allowing it to evolve into grief and loss. It is important to empathize with the child, that inner child who experienced the full force of the trauma. As an adult, you have a different view of what your abuse was like. Try to see it through the eyes of your inner child at whatever age you were when the abuse first began. If you find this difficult, try watching a child who is the age you were when you were first abused. Feeling the grief is hard; having someone there to share the tears makes it a little more bearable.

Stage Nine: Dealing with anger

Anger is a central component in your response to your abuse. You must acknowledge the anger you feel because of the cruelty you have experienced in your life. I believe that the inability to quell anger and rage, and deal with it in a positive way will jeopardize your potential for recovery. It is something that must be faced, but allow yourself the permission to process through this stage in slow, gentle steps. When confronting anger, survivors usually fall into two categories: rageaholics, who know nothing aside from rage and anger; or anger repressors, who stuff down the angry feelings because they see them as uncontrollable and potentially life-threatening. However, dealing with feelings of anger, rage, revenge, betrayal, and mistrust is very important. You might find yourself beginning this stage by expressing anger towards your therapist. Know that this is usually transference and is healthy. In this stage, you learn that you can let go of the anger that in the past has either been hidden away, or has erupted in unsuitable places and been considered irrational or inexplicable. You will begin to recognize what true anger is and let go of the rage that is no longer productive. Accepting true anger, while learning to express it without guilt, is an important skill to learn at this point in your recovery. Take time with this. Process your anger. Try shredding newspaper, pounding pillows, taking fast walks, expressing anger in your journal, throwing old dishes (from a secondhand store perhaps) at a brick wall to safely express your feelings.

Stage Ten: Confronting the offender(s)

Stage ten involves confronting the offender(s) and possibly non-offending family members who did not protect you or failed to respond to your needs. Let me be clear: I do not believe that face-to-face confrontation is a requirement for recovery. However, I believe that some form of confrontation is necessary. If you are set on the idea of face-to-face confrontation, please consider the following before you start: Only confront one offender at a time. Make a list of reasons why you want to confront the offender directly and what you hope to gain from this confrontation. Discuss this in detail with your therapist to ensure that you have set realistic goals and are not setting yourself up to find the idealized family again. Next, prepare a statement that you want to read to the offender, which includes everything you want to say in the meeting. Decide on a safe place to confront the offender; it should be on your turf or in neutral territory. Do not confront your offender alone; choose several support people to be with you. Finally, once you have completed the confrontation, schedule an appointment with your therapist to debrief. Get good support before, during, and after. For those who are not interested in a face-to-face confrontation, you have other options: Write a detailed letter to your offender to explain how his/her abuse has affected your life. You can choose to send it to the offender, or read it aloud to your therapist and support group. If your offender is dead, read the letter to others and then burn it in your fireplace; or write it on biodegradable paper and float it away in a river, or fly it away in a water-soluble helium balloon. You might also consider creating a ceremony to say goodbye to the idealized family.

Stage Eleven: Stabilizing emotions

In stage eleven, resurfacing memories and emotions come together and you begin to feel a stabilization in all aspects of your life. You can begin to accept your memories without feeling like they are occurring in the present and without resorting to old coping skills. Emotional healing brings with it resolution, resolve, and determination. Memories, shame, fear, guilt, anger, and other feelings no longer control your life. The feelings of panic and terror that came when you were experiencing flashbacks and flooding are now gone. Recovery work in this phase focuses less on the past, as you begin to devote more energy to the present and the future. You find that you no longer need to reenact in your adult relationships the abuse you suffered as a child. Physical symptomology related to the abuse subsides, and you begin to feel more connected to your body. The emotional, mental, and spiritual parts of yourself begin to come together for the first time since the abuse began. You may find yourself confronted by issues of self-sabotage; don't give up, you may just be feeling some apprehension about the therapeutic relationship ending or changing. Discuss this with your therapist. Know that the journey is not over, but you should be able to see the light at the end of the tunnel.

Stage Twelve: Exploring forgiveness issues

I am not only talking about forgiving your offender(s), which is optional, I am talking about forgiving yourself as well. Forgiving your offender(s), and perhaps non-offending family members who did not protect you, is a decision that is yours and yours alone. No one should tell you to do it; forgiveness must come from your heart and in your own way. If you are considering forgiving an offender or a non-offending family member, here are a few things to think about: Are you finished with the anger stage? You can only carry out forgiveness after you have dealt with all your own anger. Has the person you are forgiving accepted responsibility for the abuse? If not, what are your reasons for forgiving him/her? If you are considering telling someone you forgive them, do not attempt this until you have worked through the stages between confrontation and forgiveness. Finally, an old friend told me that you can't forgive someone until you know what you are forgiving them for. I agree with this and use it as an example for people who try to tell me that forgiveness comes first — it doesn't. To forgive yourself, you must know, in your heart of hearts, that you were not responsible for your abuse IN ANY WAY! Perhaps you felt responsible for your abuse in the past. Now is the time to forgive yourself for believing that lie. Make a list of all the things you are forgiving yourself for and create a ceremony for releasing it. Forgiving yourself should greatly decrease your personal feelings of guilt.

Stage Thirteen: Developing sexual healing

Since sexual offenders usually find pleasure in the very experience that caused their victims so much pain, you may feel confused about sex, sexuality, and intimacy. Sexual healing involves understanding and exploring what you need and what you want from sexual relationships, understanding that safe sex and sex by choice (not obligation) is as important in a relationship as the sexual act itself, reevaluating dating and sexual behaviors, feeling safe and loving towards your own body, working through sexual dysfunction issues, and coming to terms with any pleasure your body may have felt during the abuse. Many survivors go through an adolescent sexual development stage as a way to find what is right for them. This may begin with celibacy and move through friendships, flirting, embracing, touching, fondling, and exploring sexual likes and dislikes. Much of this occurs off and on throughout the recovery journey, but there will come a time when you will want to focus entirely on sexual healing. There are some wonderful books and tapes out there to help you with this process. See the suggested reading list for survivors.

Stage Fourteen: Finding spiritual healing

Sadly, most mental health professionals today do not address the spiritual component of healing. This does not mean, however, that it is not an important part of recovery. For many survivors, especially those who experienced ritual abuse, spirituality may have been something that was tainted as part of their abuse. Finding spiritual healing is especially difficult for those who were abused as a form of religious worship, abused by someone from their church, abused by people who adhered to a specific religion, and/or who told someone from their church but were not believed. However, each person has a spiritual element in her/his life that needs to find peace and centeredness. I am not speaking specifically of organized religion, but more of a consciousness, an essence or an inner vitality. You may be in touch with your spiritual self when you are in a church, temple or synagogue, or maybe you find it in nature, holding a child, watching a sunset, listening to beautiful music, dealing with issues of birth and death, and making a connection with good things that have happened in your past. I believe that everyone has a silver thread in their life, someone or something that allowed them to survive the pain, cruelty, and awfulness of the abuse and still evolve into the wonderful and unique person they are. If you are new to this journey, you may have read the last sentence and said, "There is nothing wonderful and unique about me." But there is, my friend, and you will find it if you stay on this path of recovery. Getting in touch with your silver thread will reaffirm your worth and bring joy to your life. Spiritual healing comes from within; it is the very core of who you are, and it is possible. (If you are interested in sharing your spiritual healing journey, see "Invitation to Authors" located in the back of this book.)

Stage Fifteen: Realizing peace within

Taking control of your life, becoming more present and future-oriented allows you to focus on your plans, goals, dreams, and wishes for tomorrow. You now realize there is a peace within. Now you are able to integrate the experiences of your life and realize who you have become. You are now able to see your abuse as something that occurred in the past. While it will affect your present life, it does not control it. You can now behave in self-protective ways, using boundaries, anger, communication, assertiveness, and self-defense skills to remove yourself from the victim role. You have passed through the victim mentality to survivor and you are now a thriver. Celebrate this growth! It was hard work, but you persevered and made it. Communicate what this path has been for you to other survivors who are on the path behind you. It is often hard to know that there is hope when you are in the midst of flooding and anger. While you cannot do the work for others, you can share your personal experiences. You have given yourself a wonderful gift: a complete life. Celebrate!

DEALING WITH
FLASHBACKS OR FLOODING

When flashbacks or flooding occur, many survivors do not know how to deal with the intensity of their feelings. During the first week of treatment I give my clients a homework assignment: Develop an emergency list that tells you how to take care of yourself in times of flashbacks, flooding or a crisis. The list should contain ten to fifteen items.

I encourage clients to carry their lists with them at all times and to have them posted in prominent places throughout their homes, workplaces, and cars. When flashbacks occur, and they will, go through the list as many times as you need to de-escalate the feelings. Some people need a second list of activities that they can do in their work setting, so be sure to prepare for that. Here are some things you might want to put on your list:

1. Sit up straight with your feet flat on the floor. Inhale through your nose, count to ten, and exhale slowly through your mouth. Repeat five times.

2. Find a safe place to be with your feelings.

3. Talk about what you are experiencing with someone who is really listening and is not afraid to ask questions.

4. Remind yourself that you are safe. Tell yourself that you are remembering what happened in the past and that you are in the present — safe.

5. Journal: Write down what you saw, how it felt, and what you are currently feeling.

6. Tell yourself that you are not going crazy. Flashbacks are part of the healing process. They are not going to make you crazy, even though it feels that way.

7. Do three things on your self-care list.

8. Do something physical, such as walking or running in place, pounding your fists on a pillow, or shredding newspaper.

9. Call someone in your support system. This may be someone from group, a recovery partner or an intimate partner. If your support person is not available, try calling a local crisis line for support.

10. Ground yourself with an object of empowerment and safety. (Many of my clients carry a special rock that they can hold onto to ground themselves.)

11. If you have gone through this list three times and are still feeling intense emotions related to flooding, flashbacks or a personal crisis, put a call in to your therapist. It is likely that your therapist will not be available the moment you call. Keep working through your list until you feel better and/or your therapist calls back.

SELF-CARE:
Learning To Love, Nurture,
And Care For Yourself

Self-care is one of the hardest tasks for a survivor. Many feel that they do not deserve to be taken care of because they are "awful," " bad," or "rotten." However, self-care is a skill you must learn early if your recovery process is to progress. The reality is, if you did not get healthy emotional or physical care as a child, no one is going to be able to meet your true inner needs now except *you*. No one — not a lover, spouse, friend, neighbor or even a therapist — is going to meet your needs the way you need them to be met. Others can help you in this process, but all will fall short of your needs and expectations. You must learn this painful truth, and begin to love, nurture, and care for yourself.

At first this may seem extremely difficult. I encourage clients to create a list of things they will do to take care of themselves during the time they are in therapy with me. The goal is to do one or two caring things for yourself every day. In the beginning this may seem foreign, but it soon becomes rote, and you begin to care for yourself — because you are someone special and because you deserve it. The following is a list of self-care suggestions compiled from suggestions from my clients. Some of these ideas may not be right for you because they may contain triggers, so be sure to make your own list.

- Take a long, hot bubble bath, listen to classical music, or light candles.

- Read a special book — not one for school, work, parenting or therapy — one just for you.

- Watch old movies, eat popcorn, and drink warm tea.

- Play with your animals; they give unconditional love.

- Reduce your expectations of yourself.

- Invest in relationships when you feel most like withdrawing.

- Focus on the present. You cannot cope with the burden of the past and the fear of the future all the time.

- Listen to special music selected just for your self-care time.
- Spend an entire day doing just what you want.
- Allow yourself to cry when you need to.
- Accept that you can't control everything.
- Take a nap.
- Go to the ocean and walk on the beach.
- Get a massage. When that is too hard, get a manicure or a pedicure.
- Go window shopping.
- Cuddle with a friend, making sure they realize it is not sexual touching.
- Allow yourself to verbalize your anger in a way that will not be destructive to yourself or others.
- Set the table with your best dishes, linen, and silver when you are having dinner by yourself.
- Write special letters to long-lost friends. Use a special pen and stationery for this.
- Lie on the couch curled up with a warm blanket, a favorite stuffed animal, and soft music.
- Eat and sleep according to a regular schedule.
- Try not to resist the recovery process because that will make you feel more alone and out of control.

BENEFITS OF GROUP THERAPY

All of my professional life, people have asked me, "What kind of therapy really works?" My response has always been the same: group therapy. I firmly believe that if you want to get a good foot-hold on your recovery, get involved in a specialized group. Sexual abuse is about secrecy. Carrying such a secret for years and years, the survivor inevitably develops a sense of isolation and a belief that she/he is different from everyone else. Many survivors also feel guilt and shame. Group therapy relieves the feelings of isolation and helps you to realize that you are not alone in your struggle.

Why group therapy?

In a group, members develop new friendships, experience emotional support, and try out new skills. The purpose of group is to help you to:

- Tell your story, be heard, and believed.
- Learn how the abuse of power and the exploitation of your body affected your life.
- Understand the shame and guilt you feel.
- Explore your personal messages about your responsibility for the abuse you suffered.
- Empower you to reclaim what was taken from you as a result of abuse.
- Become aware of your family life during childhood.
- Understand and express the losses you have experienced as a survivor of sexual abuse.

Group therapy as a tool for recovery

While group can be very scary, it can also be very helpful. Here are some thoughts from some of my clients about group therapy as a tool for recovery:

"The benefits of group therapy are peer acceptance and support. I value the opportunity to identify with others' experience and use my experience to help others."

"Group therapy is awesome! I have been through three groups and have really built a relationship with the members. Group therapy provides an outlet for venting feelings in a safe place where there are other sexual abuse survivors. It is important to be around other survivors to remind myself that I am not the only one."

"Group therapy is a good tool for recovery because you understand that other people have similar feelings, so you don't feel weird or crazy. You also learn how others cope and grow. I like seeing lots of new perspectives."

"After you get over the scary part, the feelings of 'oneness' are amazing. You don't feel so alone when you are in a group."

"I think group helped me to have more compassion for myself. I have worked towards liking myself and trying not to worry about other people and their feelings. I found out that I am not such a horrible person after all."

"Because of group I am more positive about myself. I now know that I am not alone and I am believed. I am not scared of being crazy or that I might 'go away' permanently. I can do anything."

Finding the right group

During my time as a counselor, I have developed fifteen different types of groups for survivors of sexual abuse. I break them into three different levels of recovery:

Level One: These groups are for survivors who have either never been in a group or are just beginning their recovery journey. This group is highly structured and allows time for participants to gain information and work on common issues.

Level Two: These groups are only recommended for those who have been involved in a structured group setting. This type of group is less structured and allows ample time for individual problem solving.

Level Three: These groups are what most people would call a "process-oriented" group. These groups are more flexible, allowing for group decision-making, and include material of an advanced nature.

When selecting a group, I encourage you to decide where you fit in these levels and to search for a group that meets your specific needs. You might find yourself wanting to jump into a level three group right away, but I find that starting with structure, while frustrating, lays a good foundation for recovery work.

What to look for in a group

There are a lot of groups out there. Here are some things to consider before you join one:

- Every group, except nonfacilitated self-help groups, should require a face-to-face group screening. This is a time to meet the facilitator(s), find out what type of group it is, and ask all the questions you want. Group screenings are helpful because they are an opportunity for the facilitators to screen out people who are not ready for group or do not have the right personality for a group process.

- You should know, preferably in writing, what the commitments, goals, and purposes of the group are before you start.

- I believe that if you get involved with a group, you and the other participants should be willing to make a written commitment to attend the group for a pre-set number of sessions.

Messages for those just starting group

At the completion of every group, I have my clients answer the following question: "Suppose you were just beginning group tonight. What would you have liked to know then that you know now? Write a message to those who will be starting group in the future." Here are some of their responses:

"I know you might be very scared, but you are not really living until you begin the healing process."

"It is really scary at first, but know that your group members and the group meetings will become the most important part of the week."

"What you put into group is what you will get out of it! Even though at times it gets really rough, it always gets better and that means you are one step closer to peace of mind."

"The healing process is gradual, but the changes are so important."

"It is vital to share your pain and not to try to do it alone."

"Group is a warm place to deal with the issues of the past. Remember, it takes more energy to deny how this is affecting your life than to deal with it."

"This may be the most agonizing and the most joyful journey of your life. Hang on!"

"Look at the faces of your group members and know that they will accept you and honor you no matter how ugly your abuse was and no matter how ashamed you are of it. You will be loved. You are important."

A final thought

While group is not for everyone, I believe it is the best answer for the majority of survivors. If you are in individual therapy, discuss seeking out a group to augment your current treatment with your therapist. Although individual and group therapy together may be a financial burden, it really is an excellent combination.

SEARCHING FOR
SOMEONE TO TRUST

Perhaps the most difficult stumbling block in an adult victim's recovery from childhood incest and abuse is the lack of someone to trust — someone who will be there through the thick and thin of recovery and who will rejoice when it is time to be free to fly with your own wings. The struggle and search for this type of support system can leave one feeling rejected, hopeless, and alone.

While we commend the support that is rapidly growing for children who have been victimized, there continues to be little assistance for adult victims, who search for some sort of "normalcy" within their lives. As the years pass, and the secret gets forced deeper and deeper into the victim's inner core, the ability to open up and trust someone is much more difficult to develop. However, there comes a time, whether today or next year, when the secret within cries to be let out. Then begins the search for someone to trust.

The purpose here is to give some specific guidelines for this process of finding someone to trust. It is more conducive to recovery to spend time and energy on healing rather than on searching for a therapist. The following case study is an example of the trials one adult victim of child sexual abuse had to go through to get the help she so desperately needed.

Sara: A case study

Sara, a victim of multiple abuses from her earliest years, had gotten to a point where she was no longer able to separate the past from the present. Everything that went on in her life as an adult reminded her of the past she kept trying to forget.

She had no memory of the abuses that tormented her for many years; they were merely "nightmares" or "clouded images" that she didn't relate to any personal life experiences. Continual mood swings left her suicidal, self-destructive, frustrated, angry, repulsed, and disgusted. She had forgotten how to cry, laugh, and live . . . if she ever really knew. She hid within a world that she alone had created and feared leaving her home to do even the simplest chores. Trapped, she panicked and felt that she would no longer be able to go on.

Sara had unconsciously been looking for someone to whom she could tell her secret for many, many years. She remembered more than once being called into the vice-principal's office for misbehaving in school. But no one ever asked, no one ever heard the internal cries of a ten-year-old girl, and she didn't know how to put into words what was really going on in her life. "Dad touches me where he shouldn't," or "Grandfather makes me kiss him funny when I sit on his lap." No one ever saw the signs that were written on her face.

At age twelve, Sara's mother took her to a psychiatrist at the request of the school. He told her that they would be good friends as he started to make advances toward her.

Her first year in college — 3,000 miles away from home — Sara tried to kill herself. She was shuffled off to the confines of the university medical center, where she was asked a lot of questions, given a couple of tests, and never, never once, asked why she tried to do it.

Later that year in another attempt to kill herself, Sara first called the college hotline. She spoke with the director of the counseling center, who encouraged her to come over and talk. They talked, and he listened sensitively, and quickly referred her to another counselor. With this person she spent two years talking about why she hated school, why she couldn't stand her roommates, and her dreams of marriage to a knight on a white horse who would make everything better. After two years of this she was referred to a local mental health clinic because, as the therapist said, "I couldn't deal with the slowness of Sara's pace in therapy. We never seemed to work a problem through without having to go back to the beginning and work through it all over again."

An additional two years were spent with a psychiatrist talking about her "avoidance of sexual discussions," as he put it. By this time she had gone through three different types of group therapy, focusing on a variety of nonrelated topics, including assertiveness, socialization, and women's issues. Never once in her entire time in therapy did anyone ever mention sexual abuse. Sara's problem was variously diagnosed as depression, borderline personality disorder, manic-depression, psychosis, hysteria, and myriad other catch-all phrases.

One morning after three months of a never-ending roller coaster ride on drugs and alcohol, mixed with confusion, self-mutilating behavior, and personal turmoil, Sara realized she could not take the volcano that was building inside her any more. Making a "planned escape," Sara began to swallow the pills she had stored away in vitamin bottles for some time. This escape had been long planned in fine detail, but never completely carried out, "Until today," she thought. There seemed to be no way out but death. The future looked hopeless, and Sara didn't know how to go on with the facade of living any more.

Before passing out, Sara called a local women's hotline, and they saw that she was taken to the emergency room of a nearby hospital. Released four hours later, she returned home with nothing accomplished and no one to take care of her.

It was at this point, in a moment of clarity, that Sara realized she had to find someone to trust. She made a list of what she wanted out of her life, her marriage, her world, and she decided that no matter how long it would take, or how frightening it would be, she would go in search of someone who could help her find the answers to her life's questions. Being a person who believed in prayer, she prayed for God to provide her with a solution, someone to listen, someone to learn from, someone with whom she could share.

Sara found that person. After years of searching frantically for life and help she found someone ready to listen. She found a therapist who would support her and allow her to grow, building trust at a pace that she could handle. But life had just begun. Still there were the suicidal intentions, and the multitude of feelings she had to confront. After watching and working with her for more than a year and a half, her therapist finally asked, "Sara, have you ever been sexually abused?" And then the work really began. But she had, at last, found someone to work with her, someone to trust, someone to show her the reasons to go on, and someone to fight for her.

The point of this case study is that counseling cannot merely focus on one aspect of the client, such as acting-out behavior, self-abuse, or suicidal thoughts. A therapist has to be willing to look beyond all of that and see the person as a whole — the whole body, mind, and spirit.

While each client-counselor partnership is different and unique, there are some basic qualities inherent in all therapists who have the potential to become someone to trust. Some points to remember:

Look for someone with experience

The length and extent of the therapist's education is not a major factor. Anyone with a Ph.D., M.S., or pastoral counseling degree is just as qualified to work on the variety of topics needing exploration as someone with an M.D. The only significant difference, besides salary, status, and counseling theories, is that an M.D. may directly prescribe medications, whereas other therapists must rely on the occasional support of physicians for medical management of drugs.

What is important is that the counselor you see has expertise that relates to you and your problems. Check out specific counselors by getting referrals from people you feel you can trust. People who have been through similar experiences can offer valuable insights.

Trust yourself

Call and make an intake appointment with the therapist you have chosen. Go trusting your own intuition and gut-level feelings to let you know whether or not this is someone you can work with. You are your own best indicator. Use this time to meet the counselor, discuss basic issues you would be interested in working on, and "interview" him or her. Be prepared to ask specific questions that may be pertinent to you, i.e., cost, personal beliefs, type of training in certain areas of expertise, what rules the therapist adheres to in the course of therapy. You have the right to answers delivered in a straightforward and honest manner. Remember, you are commissioning the counselor to join in your journey toward recovery.

After the session, allow yourself time to think. Is this someone you could work with in the closeness of a therapeutic relationship?

Do they seem preoccupied, or do they present a manner that makes you feel comfortable and safe? Do they have patience? Is the therapist humble, having the ability to learn, while being confident in his/her own skills? Is there room for play within the course of therapy, and does the therapist have a good sense of humor? Are they willing to be there for you during times of crisis for phone calls and/or extra-session time if needed?

Do not feel bound to return to a counselor just because you feel the person was nice to you, or that you have to take care of the counselor's needs. Remember, you are there to work on your own issues. If you feel trapped into meeting their needs and "getting well" for them, the time spent in therapy will be lost. It is quite easy for adult victims of abuse to fall back into the caretaking roles they were placed in when the original abuse occurred.

Seek empathy

One of a therapist's most important qualities is the ability to respond with empathy. This does not mean they have to have shared the same life experiences, but they must be able to understand how you feel — as if they were you. Then they can come to a full understanding of the problem and work from a more objective view when it comes to problem solving.

It is very important that the therapist be willing to self-disclose and share some of their own life experiences with the client. These experiences help the therapist relate to where the client is emotionally at the time, while providing a different view of understanding for the client. Allowing a time of open, honest, genuine sharing is an indication that a counselor is trustworthy.

Establish communication

There should always be active communication between client and therapist. Modern counseling is a two-way process. If something is not working, be willing to tell your therapist, and search together for a means to get things moving again. Both counselor and client must be flexible so that the best therapy is obtained for the client.

Develop support structures outside of therapy

Rarely does the counseling session truly end when the client walks out of the office. There are always more thoughts to deal with and feelings to be discussed. It is very important that the client go about developing positive support structures outside of therapy. This type of support can be especially helpful when dealing with emotionally charged topics. Surround yourself with people who, while they might not know the whole picture, have some idea of what is going on in your life and are willing to give unconditional support and care. Therapy is emotionally draining, and the better your support system, the sooner you will recover.

Often, group therapy in conjunction with individual counseling provides this much needed supportive atmosphere. Within a group setting, you can begin to establish outside support systems with others who will be able to relate to your experiences and understand and validate your struggles.

Make your decision for recovery

Once you have found a therapist you can trust, you must make the decision that you are ready and willing to work on your own issues. The courage to take this step does not come easily. It often appears that the risks involved in opening yourself to healing far outweigh the advantages. You will have to grapple with fears of change, processing through pain, and the implications of recovery for family and friends. It will take all your willingness to grow and stretch yourself through constant self-examination. The process toward healing may seem slow, tedious, and tiresome; it will be intermingled with periods of self-doubt, denial, and fear. However, the rewards are worth it all: recovery!

SURVIVOR'S REACTIONS

The following material on victims' reactions is presented in a generalized format. However, I caution you not to look at all this information as either dark or light, with no shades of gray. Life isn't that way. Every assault situation was a real event; if you were the victim, it has left its mark on you, as a child and as an adult. The worst response to this material would be to say, "After reading this I guess my experience wasn't that big of a deal, so what am I making all the fuss about?" I repeat, if it happened to you, it happened 100 percent.

How children react

A child victim's reaction to sexual assault depends several factors:

1. What is the relationship between the child and the molester? The closer the molester is to the child and the family unit, the greater the trauma. If the molester is a total stranger, the long-term effects will be less.

2. How many times did the sexual assault occur? The greater the number, the greater the trauma. A single assault seems to be easier for a child to deal with than multiple assaults over a long period of time.

3. How much force or violence was used on the child during the assault? Again, the more violent the attack, the greater the child's emotional reaction to the assault.

4. Was emotional abuse — especially shame, guilt, and/or embarrassment — used as a tactic to sexually assault the child? The answer to this question is almost always yes, and this results in greater emotional reactions and longer-term effects on the child.

The amount of trauma the child experienced can be directly related to these and perhaps other issues. Child victims of sexual assault may be expected to exhibit any or all of the following negative reactions: sleep and eating problems, fear of school, emotional regression, depression, suicidal thoughts (yes, even in children!), physical symptomology, shock, and bedwetting.

Comments from adult incest victims

Many people do not realize the long-lasting effects incest can have on children. Even into adulthood, victims carry a plethora of very intense feelings. The same negative reactions that were listed for children can persist into their adult lives. For many, the trauma of their abuse has been buried away even to the point of forgetting that it ever happened. When this occurs, the symptoms are the same, but no one can put all the pieces together. Only after the nightmares of the abuse are confronted can recovery take place.

The following is a list of some of the feelings victims typically experience and some of the comments that accompany these feelings:

1. Loss of control: "My whole life is falling apart. Why am I so powerless?" or "I need someone to put me back together again."

2. Loss of feelings: "I don't feel anything, I am numb"; or "I think I have forgotten how to cry."

3. Fear: "I know I am not safe, he is going to come back and get me again." "I think I am going crazy." "The nightmares I have overwhelm me"; or "Is it ever going to be the way it was before all this happened?"

4. Anxiety: "I can't breathe, I am really nervous." "I just want to eat and eat and eat." "I can't go outside anymore; it really scares me to be there"; or "I feel like my stomach is all tied up in knots."

5. Anger: "I hate him so very much, I could just kill him." "All men are alike, the only thing they want you for is sex"; or "I feel like Mt. St. Helens is going to erupt inside me at any moment."

6. Denial: "I was lying, nothing really happened." "What happened to me wasn't that big a deal." "I just made the whole thing up"; or "I was just lying to get some attention."

7. Confusion: "I don't really know what happened to today, it just kind of disappeared." "I'm feeling overwhelmed and having trouble focusing on my day-to-day chores"; or "It seems like the abuse just happened today, when I really know it happened long ago."

8. Depression: "I am doing nothing but crying all the time." "Everything is just hopeless, I'm too tired to fight this anymore"; or "I think about killing myself every day!"

9. Helplessness: "I can't do what you expect me to do, I am just not capable."

10. Self-mutilation: "I feel like I need to cut myself just to release the tension that builds up inside of me. Once I have cut, things seem to feel a whole lot better."

11. Shame: "I have to take five showers a day and wash my hands hundreds of times, because I feel so dirty."

12. Guilt: "I just know it was all my fault. Maybe if I had done something different it would never have happened"; or "He told me he had to do it because I was so very, very bad. I should have been a better child."

A P P E N D I X

SUGGESTED RESOURCES FOR ADULT SURVIVORS OF CHILDHOOD SEXUAL ABUSE

Books

The Right to Innocence:
Healing the Trauma of Childhood Sexual Abuse
Engel, Beverly. Los Angeles: Jeremy Tharcher, Inc., 1989. An inexpensive paperback that provides a wealth of knowledge for survivors starting the recovery process. Especially helpful are the "Exercises for Saying Good-bye" for survivors who are "divorcing" their offending parents.

Growing Beyond Abuse:
A Workbook For Survivors Of Sexual
Exploitation or Childhood Sexual Abuse
Nestingen, Singe L., M.A.; Lewis, Laurel Ruth. Minneapolis: Omni Recovery, 1991. A remarkable book for survivors at every level of their personal recovery. This workbook uses recovery readings, journal writing, art therapy, and spiritual expression as recovery tools. Topics include denial, trust, anger, self-esteem, sexuality, and grief. Each step of the way the reader is given a variety of options for exercises to promote healing. The excellent resource list at the end of this book is an additional bonus. To place an order, write to: Omni Recovery, Inc., P.O. Box 50033, Minneapolis, MN 55403.

Adults Molested as Children:
A Survivor's Manual for Women and Men
Bear, Evan with Dimock, Peter T. Seattle: The Safer Society Press, 1989. A helpful manual written for and by survivors.

Secret Survivors:
Uncovering Incest and Its Aftereffects in Women
Blume, Sue E. New York: John Wiley and Sons, 1990. This book
has been a helpful recovery tool for many of my clients. It focuses
on what incest does to those who survive it. Most helpful is the
view of empowerment in the healing process. Blume has created
an "Aftereffects Checklist" which is helpful for survivors and therapists alike.

My Father's House: *A Memoir of Incest and of Healing*
Fraser, Sylvia. New York: Ticknor and Fields, 1988. This book does
an outstanding job of demonstrating a child's desire to survive and
the great lengths to which the mind will go to increase the prob-
ability of survival. *My Father's House* pointedly shows the child's
need to be loved, the simultaneous fear of and desire for discovery,
and the incredible amount of confusion experienced by a child in
abusive circumstances. Fraser includes a compelling portrait of the
overwhelming guilt and responsibility felt by the child. This book,
unlike others, graphically depicts the painful path of recovery. The
discussion includes denial, restlessness, nightmares, the horror at
the realization of what happened, anger, hate, the need to tell, and
lastly, the need to forgive and love not only Daddy but, most impor-
tantly, the child within. A survivor myself, I was deeply touched by
this story. This is an excellent book. I would recommend it to both
survivors and those attempting to understand and/or love a survivor. — Reviewed by P. Wickham

Secret Shame: *I Am A Victim Of Incest*
Janssen, Martha. Minneapolis: Augsburg Fortress, 1991. A painful
yet joyous poetic commentary on one survivor's personal healing
process. Completely in verse, this book takes the reader through
the author's preschool years to her healing. Janssen provides a real
sense of hope for those who are suffering.

Recovering From Sexual Abuse And Incest
Gust, Jean; Sweeting, Patricia. Bedford, Massachusetts: Mills and
Sanderson, 1992. The authors have adapted the Twelve Steps of

Alcoholics Anonymous for survivors of sexual abuse. Each chapter includes an explanation of the process of working the step, including personal examples, followed by questions designed to help the reader identify feelings and experiences. The spiritual aspects of recovery are explained broadly enough so that most readers will find something to which they can relate. Survivors who are new to the twelve-step program of recovery, as well as those who are already active in a program, will find this book a helpful supplement to their recovery. — Reviewed by LSM

Women's Sexuality After Childhood Incest
Westerlund, Elaine, Ph.D. New York: W.W. Norton & Co., 1992. The first thing I liked about this book was the absence of euphemisms in its title. It is the kind of book I like to read on a bus and watch how people react. The second thing I appreciated is that the author, a psychologist, is also an incest survivor. Although the book is highly research-oriented, anecdotal findings are included, as well as specific implications for therapy. Westerlund covers central themes related to body perception, sexual preference, functioning, and lifestyle. As an incest survivor, I've often found myself on the outside looking in, when comparing myself to others with similar feelings and experiences. Behaviors less openly discussed, even among survivors, such as self-mutilation, are identified and sensitively explained. I found the highly objective style of Westerlund's reporting to be useful when identifying issues that often feel too emotionally charged to process. Westerlund's research can have only positive implications for the future health and well-being of survivors. This is good reading for individuals in the recovery process and essential for professionals working with survivors. — Reviewed by LSM

Reclaiming The Heart:
A Handbook of Help and Hope for Survivors of Incest
McClure, Mary Beth. New York: Warner Books, 1990. Another quality paperback especially recommended for those just beginning the process of recovery. Recovery stories accompany each chapter and add a symbol of real hope for survivors.

Surviving the Wreck
Osborn, Susan. New York: Henry Holt, 1992. This book, written as a novel, deals with the issues of sexual abuse and the resounding effects on the family system. My struggle with the book is the format. While the descriptions of abuse are shocking and realistic, I worry that a novice reader would question, "Is this is just a novel? Does this really happen in real families?" The answer, of course, is yes!

When You're Ready:
A Women's Healing from Childhood
Physical and Sexual Abuse by her Mother
Evert, Kathy; Bijkerk, Inje. San Luis Obispo, California: Launch Press, 1987. Several clients who were abused by their mothers strongly recommend this volume. It is one of the few books to address mothers as offenders.

Be sure to check out additional resources in the *Partners in Healing* chapter.

Audio Tapes

The Isle Of Pleasure: *Your Path to Sexual Fulfillment*
Underwood, Judy K.; Gaynor, Pamela A. Underwood and Gaynor declare these tapes to be "a wonderful, safe way to explore and recover your sexuality." If you are ready to get in touch with your body from which you may have been detached for many years, this is must listening! I recommend it for every female survivor of sexual abuse who is at the point in her recovery where she is ready to work on reclaiming her sexuality. Many of my clients have used the tapes and found the easy pacing to be just what they needed. There is a heterosexual series and a lesbian series. The tapes are tastefully done, empowering, and give the listener the permission needed to explore her own sexuality. For more information contact: Odyssey, 1-800-733-6104.

Welcome To The World

Underwood, Judy K. According to Underwood, "This tape will create the nurturing beginning your infant self deserves. You will experience profound acceptance as a female. *Welcome to the World* uses guided imagery to welcome your younger self to a new life filled with love and caring." We use this tape in our "Finding Your Inner Child" groups, and the participants have found it to be a very powerful tool. I recommend repeated use of the tape because we have found that new feelings emerge every time the tape is played. *Welcome to the World* allows my clients to work on getting in touch with their inner child in a safe way, between therapy sessions. For more information contact: Odyssey, 1-800-733-6104.

Survivor

Morgan, Pam. Soothing music for those working through their childhood sexual abuse recovery issues. Pam herself sings and creates the music. She says, "To those of you who have survived childhood abuse, I offer understanding, compassion, and hope. We are each lovable and worthwhile human beings simply because we exist, and we deserve the best that we can give ourselves." I recommend it to you all. To purchase the tape write: Pam Morgan, 1610 N.E. Broadway, #539, Portland, OR 97232.

A Story of Hope

Van Derbur, Marilyn. Available on both audio and video, Van Derbur, a former Miss America and incest survivor talks about the road to recovery. This is must viewing for both survivors — especially those who are struggling with denial and an inability release their shame — and their partners. To order, write to: Marilyn Van Derbur, 195 South Dahlia St., Denver, CO 80222. For VHS send $24.00 plus $2.00 postage and handling; for audio cassette send $14.00 plus $1.50 postage and handling. Prepaid orders only.

RECOMMENDED READING
FOR PROFESSIONALS

Therapy for Adults Molested as Children: *Beyond Survival*
Briere, John. New York: Speinger Publishing Co., 1989. A well-written guide for professionals. Special focus in the areas of post-traumatic stress disorder (PTSD), borderline personality disorder, and a trauma symptom check (TSC-33) list that deserves further research findings but is quite helpful.

Healing the Incest Wound: *Adult Survivors in Therapy*
Courtois, Christine. New York: W.W. Norton & Co., 1988. Courtois, an early researcher in the field of sexual abuse recovery, reviews theories and approaches to treatment.

Psychological Trauma and the Adult Survivor:
Theory, Therapy and Transformation
McCann, Lisa; Pearlman, L. A. New York: Brunner/Mazel, 1990. Written by the developers of the McPears Belief Scale, this book pinpoints therapy issues that should be addressed with clients.

Understanding Child Sexual Abuse Maltreatment
Faller, Kathleen Coulborn. Newbery Park, California: Sage Publications, 1990. This book is largely based on research by the University of Michigan's Project on Child Abuse. Sometimes it is dry reading, but I especially like the insights on working with law enforcement and legal professionals.

Breaking Down the Wall of Silence:
The Liberating Experience of Facing Painful Truth
Miller, Alice. New York: Dutton, 1991. Miller is well known for her pioneering works on sexual abuse. This book is in the forefront of treatment today.

Treating PTSD: *Cognitive-Behavioral Strategies*
Foy, David W., editor. New York: Guilford Press, 1992. An excellent overview of the available materials on the treatment of post-traumatic stress disorder (PTSD). Especially helpful are the last two chapters for survivors of sexual abuse.

The Second Rape: *Society's Continued Betrayal of the Victim*
Madigan, Lee; Gamble, Nancy. New York: Lexington Books, 1991. The statistics about rape are stark enough: Every hour sixteen rapes are attempted and ten women are raped in the United States. It is the most under-reported crime, partly because of the second rape. The second rape is the violation that occurs when the rape survivor seeks professional help through police, medical personnel, lawyers, and even therapists. The authors give explicit details that may be upsetting to some readers. The book validates the rape survivor's experiences and sensitizes others to the lack of support presently available. With the hope that the system will be forced to change, the authors encourage women to report the crime, despite the potential of further emotional trauma. — Reviewed by LSM

READING GUIDE ON
TOPICS RELATED TO
SEXUAL ABUSE RECOVERY

Addictions (Drugs, Alcohol and Food)

Double Duty:
Help for the Adult Child Who is Also Sexually Abused
Black, Claudia. New York: Ballantine Books, 1990. Black, who is well known for her extensive writings for adult children of alcoholics, has written another excellent book. This book provides information for survivors who are dealing with their own addictions as well as a history of dysfunction in their families. Now in paperback, it is must reading for anyone doing "double duty."

Rx For Recovery:
The Medical and Health Guide for
Alcoholics, Addicts, and Their Families
Weisberg, Jeffrey; Hawes, Gene. New York: Ivy Books, 1990. An excellent book that examines issues not covered elsewhere: medications and their impact on recovery, handling common problems like pain, sleeplessness, and dental care, and how family members can assist the recovering addict.

When Food Is Love:
Exploring the Relationship Between Eating and Intimacy
Roth, Geneen. New York: Dutton, 1991. While I think all of Roth's books are excellent, I like this one the best. I also use it for clients without eating issues because of the honest and clear information that is given about relationships. This is one of those books you can not put down.

Codependency

Love Is A Choice: *Recovery For Codependent Relationships*
Hemfelt, Robert; Minith, Frank; Meier, Paul. Nashville: Thomas
Nelson Publishers, 1991. Using numerous examples, the book
identifies ten traits of codependency, followed by a ten-stage recovery process including 1) exploration and discovery, 2) relationship
history/inventory, 3) addiction control, 4) leaving home and saying
goodbye, 5) grieving your loss, 6) new self-perceptions, 7) new
experiences, 8) reparenting, 9) relationship accountability,
10) maintenance. The recovery principles are written from a Christian perspective. — Reviewed by LSM

Codependent No More:
How to Stop Controlling Others and Start Caring for Yourself
Beattie, Melody. New York: Harper and Row, 1987. This was, and
is, a groundbreaking book on the subject of codependency. The
most important part of this book for survivors is "The Basics of Self
Care." Because so many survivors do not know how to care for
themselves, this is a very helpful book.

Beyond Codependency and Getting Better all the Time
Beattie, Melody. New York: Harper and Row, 1989. A follow-up to
the above-mentioned book that discusses how the author achieved
her new life. *Beyond Codependency* discusses how to move beyond
codependency and find reality.

Depression

Feeling Good: *The New Mood Therapy*
Burns, David. New York: Signet Books, 1980. While this book may
be a few years old, it is still my first choice for helping clients work
through their depression. There are a variety of tests, inventories,
and wonderful exercises to assist you in working through depression issues.

Intimacy

The Dance of Intimacy:
A Women's Guide to Courageous Acts
of Change in Key Relationships
Herner, Harriet Goldhor. New York: Harper and Row, 1989. This book is written by the author of *Dance of Anger*. It is wonderfully written, easy to read, and teaches us all some invaluable lessons.

Journaling

At A Journal Workshop:
The Basic Text and Guide for Using the Intensive Journal
Progoff, Ira. New York: Dialogue House, 1975. This book was written for people who wanted to take an "intensive journal" workshop from Progoff but were not able to. It provides ideas for setting up a journal and discusses some of the author's principles on journaling.

Shame

Uncovering Shame:
An Approach Integrating Individuals and their Family Systems
Harper, James; Hoopes, Margaret. New York: W.W. Norton & Co., 1990. While this book is not exclusively for abuse survivors, it is an excellent manual for professionals working with shame-based clients.

Abuse by Members of the Clergy

Lead Us Not Into Temptation:
Catholic Priests and the Sexual Abuse of Children
Berry, Jason. New York: Doubleday, 1992. *Lead Us Not Into Temptation* is a detailed account of child abuse in the Catholic Church and reveals how bishops have stonewalled parents and authorities, while recycling offenders.

Recovery Quilts

For the last four years, Echoes Network Counseling Center has been creating recovery quilts with pieces made by our clients. While this will never reach the magnitude of the AIDS quilts, I would like to invite you to send us your quilt square for inclusion in future recovery quilts. To date, we have three giant quilts, and they are all as wonderful and unique as the people whose squares are included in them. I take these quilts to the workshops and training sessions I do across the country, and each time I display them, participants are impacted by the emotional power sewn into them.

If you are interested in sending a quilt square to us, here are some guidelines: Squares must be ten inches in diameter *without batting* (we do that later). There needs to be a seam allowance of five-eighths of an inch on all sides of the square. Use any medium you like to decorate your square: fabric paints, stitching, transfers, piecing, batik, etc. You many include your first name on the square if you wish. Try to focus on the theme "What recovery looks like for me." Send your piece and a three-by-five-inch card with your name and address. Please specify if you want to be included in the sexual abuse, ritual abuse, MPD, or partners recovery quilt. Yes, there will be one for each! If you would like a picture of your quilt piece after it's been sewn into the entire quilt, please send $1.00 and a self-addressed, stamped envelope. Your picture will be sent as soon as the quilt is completed.

Send to:

Echoes Network Inc.
Recovery Quilts
P.O. Box 13715
Portland, OR 97213-0715

INVITATION TO
AUTHORS AND ARTISTS

If you are interested in sharing some of your experiences, feelings, and accounts of your recovery process — whether you are a survivor of sexual abuse, ritual abuse, MPD, a male survivor or the partner of a survivor — for use in future publications by Echoes Network Inc., please follow the guidelines for submissions below. We are always seeking stories, poems, and black ink drawings to use in our quarterly newsletter *SOUNDINGS* or future books on abuse recovery.

Send your writings detailing your activities to continue your personal and spiritual recovery. I am especially interested in writings on spiritual recovery issues. Be sure to indicate what your religion or viewpoint is. I am also looking for writing from partners in healing: writings by and for those living or working with survivors of sexual abuse, including therapist's insights.

Please keep in mind that I cannot personally respond to your letters without a self-addressed, stamped envelope.

Guidelines for Submissions

1. Please type or print your work. Include your name and address on each page.

2. If possible, send your material on a 3.5-inch disc, Macintosh Microsoft Word 3.0 to 5.0. **OR** IBM-compatible, 360K, 5.25-inch disc, Word Perfect 5.1.

3. One entry per page.

4. Limit of ten submissions per quarter.

5. Realize that no work will be returned. Please make copies of the material you send.

6. Include a progress report with your work. This is statement about you, your recovery (if applicable), and how you are doing today. Work without progress reports is less likely to be evaluated for publication.

7. Please be aware that you retain the copyright for your original work. Echoes Network Inc. retains the copyright to your work as it appears in the publication, including context or editorial commentary.

8. We do not identify offenders. Please use initials or pseudonyms.

9. We may edit your material for content and clarity. Include a self-addressed stamped envelope if you wish to be notified and give final approval of these changes (other than spelling, syntax, and grammar corrections).

10. We need a signed "Release to Print" statement from EVERY contributor. Please copy the one below and send it along with your submission.

Release to Print

I, _____ , have enclosed material for possible publication in future writing projects of Echoes Network Inc. I understand that by sending material, I am giving permission to print my work. I realize that my writings may be edited for content and space availability. Echoes Network Inc. and its staff are not responsible for liability due to the printing of my work. For legal reasons and for my protection, I understand that only first names and a last initial **OR** a first initial and last name **OR** a pseudonym **OR** Anonymous, will be used to identify my work.

☐ Please print my name after my work.

Print as: _____

☐ I choose not to have my name used.

☐ Please notify me of any changes to my material other than spelling, syntax or grammar. I have included a SASE.

I have read and understand the aforementioned statements:

Signed: _____ Date: _____

Send to:
Echoes Network Inc.
Editorial Review
P.O. Box 13715, Portland, OR 97213-0715

BIBLIOGRAPHY

Bliss, E. L. " Multiple Personalties." In *Archives of General Psychiatry*, vol. 37, 1388-1400, 1984.

Bliss, E. L. *Multiple Personality Disorder, Allied Disorders, and Hypnosis*. New York: Oxford University Press, 1986.

Braun, B. *Treatment of Multiple Personality Disorder*. Washington, D.C.: American Psychiatric Press, Inc., 1986.

Briere, J. *Therapy for Adults Molested as Children*. New York: Springer Publishing, Co., 1989.

Brownmiller, S. *Against Our Will*. New York: Bantam Books, 1981.

Cook, C. "Understanding Ritual Abuse: A Study of Thirty-Three Ritual Abuse Survivors." In *Treating Abuse Today*, vol. 1, issue 4, 14-19, 1991.

Coons, P. "The Differential Diagnosis of Multiple Personality Disorder: A Comprehensive Review." In *Psychiatric Clinics of North America,* vol. 7, 51-65, 1984.

Coons, P. *The Use of Patient Productions in the Diagnosis and Treatment of Patients with Multiple Personality/Dissociative States*. (Cassette recording no. kla-436-88). Alexandra, Washington: Audio Transcripts, Ltd., 1988.

Driscoll, L. N., and Wright, C. "Survivors of Childhood Ritual Abuse: Multi-generational Satanic Cult Involvement." In *Treating Abuse Today*, vol. 1, issue 4, 5-13, 1991.

Finkelhor, D. *Child Sexual Abuse: New Theory and Treatment*. New York: The Free Press, 1984.

Finkelhor, D. "Response Paper." Presented at the National Symposium on Assessing the Impact of Sexual Abuse, Huntsville, Alabama, 1987.

Groth, A. N. *Men Who Rape: The Psychology of the Offender.* New York: Plenum Press, 1979.

Groth, A. N. "The Incest Offender." In *Handbook of Clinical Intervention and Child Sexual Abuse,* A. L. Singe, ed. Lexington, Massachusetts: D.C. Heath and Co., 1982.

Mann, D. "Sexual Abuse of Men." A lecture presented to the Portland State University Fifth Annual Conference on Sexual Abuse, Portland, Oregon, 1988.

Oppenheimer, R., Palmer, R. L., and Brandon, S. "A Clinical Evaluation of Early Abusive Experiences in Adult Anorexic and Bulemic Females: Implications for Preventive Work in Childhood." Paper presented to the Fifth International Congress on Child Abuse and Neglect, Montreal, 1984.

Putman, F. W., Guroff, J. J., Siberman, E. K., Barban, L., and Post, R.M. "The Clinical Phenomenology of Multiple Personality Disorder: A review of 100 recent cases." In *Journal of Clinical Psychiatry,* vol. 47, 285-293, 1986.

Putnam, F. W. *Diagnosis and Treatment of Multiple Personality Disorder.* New York: Guilford Press, 1989.

Ross, C. A. *Multiple Personality Disorder: Diagnosis, Clinical Features and Treatment.* New York: John Wiley & Sons, 1989.

Ross, C. A., Miller, S. D., Reagor, P., Bjornson, L., Fraser, G. A., and Anderson, G. "Structures Interview Data on 102 Cases of Multiple Personality Disorder from Four Centers." In *American Journal of Psychiatry,* vol. 147, issue 5, 596-601, 1990.

Ross, C. A. "Epidemiology of Multiple Personality and Dissociation." In *Psychiatric Clinics of North America*, vol. 14, issue 3, 503-517, 1991.

Ross, C. A., Anderson, G., Fleisher, W. P., and Norton, G. R. "The Frequency of Multiple Personality Disorder Among Psychiatric Inpatients." In *American Journal of Psychiatry*, vol. 148, 12, 1717-1720, 1991.

Sedney, M. A., and Brooks, B. "Factors Associated with a History of Childhood Sexual Experiences in a Nonclinical Female Population." In *Journal of the American Academy of Child Psychiatry*, vol. 23, 215-218, 1984.

United States of America. *F.B.I. Uniform Crime Reports*. Washington, D.C., 1988.

Waldschmidt, C. "Questions and Answers." In *Psychsource*. Los Angeles: Community Psychiatric Centers, 1990.

Van Benschoten, S. C. "Multiple Personality Disorder and Satanic Ritual Abuse: The Issue of Credibility." In *Dissociation*, vol. 3, 22-30, 1990.

OTHER BOOKS BY BEYOND WORDS PUBLISHING, INC.

MEN, WOMEN AND RELATIONSHIPS:
Making Peace with the Opposite Sex
Author: Dr. John Gray
320 pages, $12.95 softbound

In a balanced and respectful way, the strengths, needs, vulnerabilities, and mysteries unique to each sex are revealed. This understanding will help the reader lower tensions, release resentments and avoid misunderstandings with the opposite sex. Outlined are strategies for successfully giving and receiving emotional support, and for creating more deeply satisfying and supportive relationships.

STRAIGHT TALK WITH YOUR GYNECOLOGIST:
How to Get Answers that Will Save Your Life
Author: Eddie Sollie, M.D., OB/GYN
246 pages, $12.95, softbound

Written in a conversational style, this how-to guide empowers women to become equal partners in their health care. Emphasizing the value of open communication, *Straight Talk* provides guidelines for choosing the best doctor for you, questions to ask your doctor before, during and after the exam and instructions for reading your own pap smear report. This book gives women the tools to take responsibility for their personal health and ask the questions that can save their lives.

AIDS-PROOFING YOUR KIDS: A Step-By-Step Guide
Authors: L. E. Acker, Ph.D.; B. C. Goldwater, Ph.D.; and
W. H. Dyson, Ph.D., M.D.
170 pages, $8.95 softbound

The first and only collection of the most practical teaching strategies currently available for educating teenagers about responsible sex. This timely book was written by three Ph.D.s who specialize in family psychology, social learning, medicine, biochemistry, and AIDS prevention. They lead parents, step-by-step, through AIDS-proofing exercises with their kids. The book gives the crucial facts on the disease and offers strategies to parents for teaching both abstinence and/or condom use.

RAISING A SON: Parents and the Making of a Healthy Man
Authors: Don and Jeanne Elium
225 pages, $18.95 hardbound, $10.95 softbound

This conversationally-styled, "how-to" book, written by family counselors, is a guide to assist both mother and father in the parts they must play in the making of a healthy, assertive, and loving man. It is suitable for parents, professional care providers and educators.

To order these books or to receive our catalog, please contact us at
Beyond Words Publishing, Inc., 13950 NW Pumpkin Ridge Rd.,
Hillsboro, OR 97123 (503) 647-5109.